Sexual Health
in Later Life

Sexual Health in Later Life

THOMAS H. WALZ
University of Iowa

NANCEE S. BLUM
University of Iowa

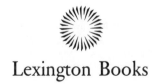

Lexington Books

D.C. Heath and Company • Lexington, Massachusetts • Toronto

Library of Congress Cataloging-in-Publication Data

Walz, Thomas H.
Sexual health in later life.

Bibliography: p.
Includes index.
1. Aged—Sexual behavior. I. Blum, Nancee S. II. Title. [DNLM:
1. Sex—in old age. 2. Sex Behavior—in old age. HQ 30 W242s]
   BF724.85.S48W35   1987   155.67   86-45932
      ISBN 0-669-14600-5 (alk. paper)
      ISBN 0-669-14599-8 (pbk. : alk. paper)

Published simultaneously in Canada
Printed in the United States of America
Casebound International Standard Book Number: 0-669-14600-5
Paperbound International Standard Book Number: 0-669-14599-8
Library of Congress Catalog Card Number: 86-45932

The paper used in this publication meets
the minimum requirements of American National Standard
for Information Sciences—Permanence of Paper
for Printed Library Materials, ANSI Z39.48-1984.

87 88 89 90 8 7 6 5 4 3 2 1

To our families

*To the success of the Gerontology Projects Program
in the School of Social Work at the University of Iowa*

*To the success of the new Geriatric Education Center
at the University of Iowa*

Contents

Acknowledgments

Special thanks are owed to the many health care professionals at the University of Iowa Hospitals and Clinics who so willingly shared their expertise on the health and treatment aspects of sexuality in the aged. The authors are especially indebted to Ian M. Smith, M.D., Director of the Geriatrics Program, Department of Internal Medicine, for his support and encouragement.

We would like to thank our many older friends and, on occasion, our patients for their candid personal insights about sexuality in later life.

1

Sexuality in the Older Adult: An Introduction

Aging is regarded as a demon that heralds approaching death, whereas sex is equated with life. That is why sexuality is especially significant for an older person's morale—it is an affirmation of life and a denial of death (Dean 1974, 136–37).

T HIS book is about sexuality in the older adult. It is written principally for older adults and for those who share in their lives. For the older adult of advanced years, these significant others often are caregivers, both the family-friend caregivers and the many professionals and paraprofessionals who work through the health, aging, and human services networks.

This book is based on three assumptions: first, barring illness or accident, most people in the United States grow to be old; second, all people are born sexual beings and remain so throughout their lives; and, third, in our present society, most people are not well prepared to understand their maturing bodies or how the aging process affects their sexual interests and capacities. The intent of this book is to correct these misunderstandings that only bring confusion and hurt to people.

There is no good way to define who is, in fact, an older adult. If you think you are one, perhaps that is the best definition. Nature does provide something of a benchmark of older adulthood for most men and for all women—the so-called change of life phenomenon. For women, of course, this is menopause, the point when the ovaries cease to function. For most men a somewhat equivalent midlife change occurs—more emotional than physical—that is referred to as the climacteric. These midlife changes are important because of their apparent relationship to our sexual physiology and hence to our ongoing sexual functioning.

This concept of older adulthood also includes a phase of advanced old age, sometimes referred to as senescence. Just when it occurs varies greatly among individuals. Chronological age is a poor measure of when old age begins. A better indication is when a person experiences the illnesses and infirmities of age. The presence of chronic disease may severely compromise one's sexuality. For this reason, our major attention will be directed to the sexuality of those of advanced years. Until recently, little was known or written about the sexual interests, needs, and functioning of people in their postretirement years.

How older adults perceive themselves as sexual beings has a lot to do with how others in their environment perceive them. We see ourselves as others see us, as the saying goes. Most women in the immediate postmenopausal phase and their middle-aged male partners are probably viewed as sexually active, although less so than younger adults. However, there is a definite societal stereotype in which those of postretirement years are assumed to be sexually retired as well. By sexually retired, we mean, of course, sexually inactive. Tragically, this stereotype is found among all classes and ages of individuals, including the elderly themselves and their professional caregivers. How many physicians have prescribed medications for elderly patients without informing them of side effects that could affect their sexual interest or capacity? How often does an activity coordinator in a nursing home fail to plan activities that promote needed "high touch" contact among residents? How often do you see a movie that treats the love between an elderly man and woman with dignity? As a culture, we do a very poor job of understanding, supporting, and promoting the sexual nature of the older adult.

We assume that older adults know how their bodies age and how this aging process may affect them sexually. To some extent, life experience is a good teacher. We do learn the facts of life more or less by muddling through them. We also know the pains of trial and error and the hazards of ignorance. Perhaps we assume that we should understand something as personal as our bodies, particularly their sexual parts, just because they are ours. Unfortunately, it does not work that way. The body is an extremely complex organism. Sexual functioning requires the full cooperation of many of its most complex systems—nervous system, circulatory system, and hormonal system. Many researchers are just beginning to understand how the body functions sexually in old age. It is easy to understand how the average older adult may be confused at times.

We sometimes forget that old age is a modern invention. Most people in human history rarely lived beyond their middle years. More women in human history have probably died in childbirth than of old age. Little wonder then that we are only now beginning to learn about sexuality in the older adult years. What might have been known, since some people have always lived to advanced old age, has been limited because of the "conspiracy of silence" about personal sexual matters. Old people rarely talked openly about their sexual feelings, needs, and activities, and others, including scientific researchers, rarely asked.

In post–World War II America, something of a sexual revolution has occurred. Sexual mores have changed. Birth control, the need to limit family size, and an intense consumer orientation have served to turn sexual expression from a simple reproduction of the species to a complex expression of love, affection, and pleasure. The human rights revolution of the 1960s included the right of control and use of our bodies. Freedom of sexual expression, including sexual preference, was part of that development. Although we tend to think this sexual revolution is felt more keenly by the young than the old, an awareness of the right to lifelong sexuality is growing among older adults.

Along with the efforts to protect women and children from sexual abuse and exploitation, we now recognize the need to protect older adults from hurtful stereotypes about being asexual in old age. It is easy to understand the need to protect vulnerable people from unwanted sexual intrusion. It is much harder to understand the violence we do to people by denying them the opportunity for sexual expression.

In this book we do not insist that older adults must be genitally sexually active (have intercourse) to be normal or happy. Whether you are sexually active or not has little bearing on your reality as a sexual being. Sexuality is something that takes place more often between the ears than between the legs. Older people have a perfect right to retire sexually, if that is their choice. Some people have successfully chosen to remain celibate their entire lives. Mahatma Gandhi, for example, made celibacy an important positive part of his life in his later years.

For those older adults who wish to remain sexually active, the need to understand how aging and their sexuality interact is essential. A lack of such basic knowledge can produce needless anxiety and can result in the drawing of false conclusions. For example, a woman who resumes sexual intercourse after a long illness could find it painful because her vagina has atrophied (become smaller). She needs to know that with a little patience it can accommodate intercourse again without pain. In another case, a man who becomes unable to obtain an erection and later is told he has diabetes needs to realize that once his diabetes is controlled, he can expect potency to return.

Except for a lucky few, illness is a common experience of advanced age. The illness, the treatment of the illness, or both, can severely affect sexual functioning. It is critical to know which changes in sexual interest and function are due to age itself and which are due to the illness or its treatment. Of course in some situations knowledge alone is not enough to restore a person to full sexual function. Changes do occur that are irreversible, although fortunately, not often. Again, we repeat, sexuality is more than just the ability to perform the gymnastics of sexual intercourse. Sexuality is closeness, intimacy, touch, caring—as much an attitude of mind as a function of the body.

As a result of the sexual revolution, perhaps the importance of genital sexuality has been oversold. All too often, sexual expression has been viewed as another product to be marketed. As we approach the topic of sexuality in the older adult, we need to remind ourselves constantly of the broader meaning and significance of our sexual nature—intercourse is only one expression of this nature.

Old age has a way of masking sexual frustrations. Since we are not expected to be sexually active in old age, the retreat from being active sexually is a step easily taken. One of the most common frustrations in old age is the loss of a sexual partner. The death or sexual retirement of one's partner can obviously complicate one's need and desire to remain a sexually active person. It is hard to tell what is more frustrating, to be expected to be sexually involved when you are not interested, or not to be sexually active when you *are* interested.

In this book we will explore what is known or accepted as fact about how the aging of the body affects sexual functioning in later life. It is important to bear in mind that the research on the subject is limited and, as with all social research, the findings are rarely 100 percent accurate. Throughout the book, we have tried to include suggestions for further reading where appropriate, and we have also included the names of self-help groups and other resources that might be helpful.

In the following chapter, we will present our own case for the benefits of continued sexual activity in old age (when and where possible). In some ways, we believe that this argument is one of the most important sections of the book. If being active sexually were not important to the well-being of the older adult, trying to improve our knowledge and understanding about the effects of aging on sexual functioning in later life would have little value.

Following the chapter about the relevance of maintaining sexual health in old age, we will talk about the physiological and biochemical changes of aging that could affect sexual functioning. The different aspects of female and male aging in this respect will be discussed.

Building on our description of the normal processes of aging as they affect sexual function, we will discuss the role that diseases and illnesses of old age may or may not play in compromising continued sexual activity. This will be followed by a chapter that explores how the treatment of chronic illness may further compromise sexual functioning in later adulthood. Ironically, the efforts to control such illness may be as devastating to sexual health as the illness itself. Again we are faced with limited knowledge of some of these disease processes and the constantly changing nature of their treatments. We need to understand that what we know today may change tomorrow.

In subsequent chapters, we will explore the psychological dimensions of how attitudes and mental states may affect sexual functioning in older adults. The mind and the emotions make important contributions to the maintenance of sexual health. This is true, of course, for individuals of all ages. All human experience may or may not become enriched with age. Sexual experience is no exception. Some can become jaded by sexual encounter and may find it hardly worth the effort. This may be the most common reason that some people go into early sexual retirement. For others, sexual activity can be a constantly growing and enriching experience. As one of our eighty-six-year-old informants reported, "I always craved sexual activity, and I still do." Love and sex have always been closely connected, and people do fall out of love as readily as they fall in love. Falling out of love makes it extremely difficult to remain sexually interested. We can fall in and out of love at any age.

There is no denying that the aging process works on both the mind and the body, and that the associated changes can take their toll on sexual vitality. Recognizing this, we have provided a chapter which discusses ways to maintain sexual health. The growing health consciousness among Americans of all ages is an encouraging sign. The physical fitness movement can only have a positive effect on improving the sexual health of those who participate.

The chapter on maintaining personal sexual health is followed by a short chapter on building sexual health into our living environments. Inasmuch as 57 percent of the elderly may call an institutional environment home at some time in their lives, and another 20 percent will experience temporary placement in such an environment, it is critical that these institutions recognize and support the sexual needs of their residents. To date, the reputation of long-term care facilities in this regard is not particularly complimentary, although some improvement has taken place in recent years.

Because the great imbalance in the numbers of men and women in later life means that many more of us may spend even more of our significant time in the company of people of our same sex, we have included a chapter about the special aspects of same sex relationships. For the aging homosexual person, this situation may be taken for granted, but for the nonhomosexual elderly person, it refocuses our views about the meaning of sexuality and aging. We also briefly explore the meaning of aging for the sexuality of gay persons with an eye to their sexual health in old age.

Returning to the issue of the need to increase our understanding of sexuality in the older adult, we thought it might be helpful if the reader could begin with a personal knowledge assessment of the subject. The following set of knowledge and attitude items were taken from the Adult Sexuality Knowledge and Attitude Test (ASKAT) developed by the authors (Walz and Blum 1986). We encourage the reader to complete the assessment and turn to appendix A of the book to check the answers. Obviously, there are no right or wrong responses to the section on attitudes. Readers may find it interesting to retake the ASKAT after reading the book.

Adult Sexuality Knowledge and Attitude Test (ASKAT)

Please answer all questions. Circle T (true) or F (false) at the right. Do not answer as you *think* you should but as you really feel.

1. The majority of persons over age sixty-five have little capacity for sexual relations. T F

2. People who have heart trouble should abstain from sexual activity because of the strain it puts on the heart. T F

3. Illness rather than age is the usual reason why an older person stops having sexual relations. T F

4. Diabetes can cause impotence in males. T F

5. The biological sexual drive in older men is considerably stronger than in older women. T F

6. Changes in sexual interest and activity in women can often be caused by the loss of female hormones (estrogen) following menopause. T F

7. Most women experience complicated physical and emotional symptoms with menopause. T F

8. Most men experience a significant loss of male hormones with their "change of life."   T   F

9. In the absence of regular sexual intercourse, the vagina of an older woman may shrink, shorten, and lose elasticity.   T   F

10. Sexual feelings may remain for the older woman, but clitoral sexual sensations generally disappear by age sixty.   T   F

11. Older women rarely masturbate.   T   F

12. Regular sexual activity appears to stimulate hormone (estrogen) production in the postmenopausal woman.   T   F

13. Since the clitoral area of older women becomes more sensitive, sexual partners need to take this into consideration during sexual relations.   T   F

14. There is a significant decrease in the production of semen in the older male.   T   F

15. Older men, unlike young men, often cannot have a follow-up erection/ejaculation within a short time after sexual intercourse.   T   F

16. Male fertility (sperm production) usually ends by age sixty.   T   F

17. Sexual activity is a good form of exercise therapy for the back, stomach, and pelvic muscles of older persons.   T   F

18. Men with prostate problems may experience diminished sexual desires.   T   F

19. An older women who continues to be sexually active will probably not be able to experience an orgasm.   T   F

20. Continued sexual activity by elderly men may led to prostate problems.   T   F

21. Impotence in older men is an expected develop-
    ment in the aging process.   T   F

22. Excessive alcohol intake in men may produce
    impotence.   T   F

23. A hysterectomy inevitably produces physical
    changes that result in diminished sexual desire in
    women.   T   F

24. Tranquilizers, antidepressants, and certain anti-
    hypertensive drugs can cause loss of sexual desire in
    men and women.   T   F

25. Toxic changes in the blood from nicotine may
    reduce sexual interest.   T   F

26. Some postmenopausal women may experience an
    increased interest in sexual intercourse.   T   F

27. Healthy men over the age of sixty have greater
    control of ejaculation than do younger men.   T   F

28. Widowhood is the most common cause of reduced
    sexual activity among older women.   T   F

29. Physical changes in the vagina of the older woman
    reduce the likelihood of pain or discomfort with
    intercourse.   T   F

30. The vagina of most older women is too fragile for
    frequent (that is, daily) sexual intercourse. T   F

31. A hysterectomy diminishes (or interferes with) a
    woman's ability to experience orgasm.   T   F

32. Regular sexual activity is the best way to maintain
    sexual functioning in later life.   T   F

33. By age seventy most men are impotent.   T   F

34. Older men are more likely to masturbate than are
    older women.   T   F

35. A man in good health can continue to father
    children throughout his lifetime.   T   F

36. Hot flashes and dizziness are unavoidable effects of
    menopause.   T   F

37. In an older man, the penis softens quickly after
    ejaculation.   T   F

38. The level of sexual interest and activity in old age
    generally parallels one's patterns of sexual interest
    and activity at a younger age.   T   F

39. For many older people, the ability to perform sex-
    ually continues long after activity ceases.   T   F

40. Older persons seldom have sexual fantasies or
    dreams.   T   F

41. Masturbation is a common way for older persons
    to obtain sexual release.   T   F

42. Older persons continue to be interested in sexual
    feelings (touch, kissing) but not in sexual
    intercourse.   T   F

43. As a man ages, it takes longer for him to achieve
    an erection.   T   F

44. Eating a big meal prior to sexual intercourse will
    stimulate sexual responsiveness in older persons.   T   F

45. A stroke is a frequent cause of impotence in men.   T   F

46. Anemia may cause diminished sexual interest in
    older women.   T   F

47. Sexual blushing (redness in the area of the ab-
    domen and breasts) is less common in older
    women than in younger women.   T   F

48. It is not uncommon for an older woman to ex-
    perience some pain with orgasm.   T   F

49. An older woman may experience shrinkage or
atrophy of the vagina in the absence of regular sexual intercourse, making any resumption of intercourse initially painful.   T   F

Please answer all questions. Remember, do not answer these as you
think you should but as you really feel. Use the number that most
closely describes the way you feel.

(1) Agree (2) Strongly Agree (3) Disagree (4) Strongly disagree

1. Masturbation by older persons is an acceptable
   method of relieving sexual tension.   ( )

2. Old men should not be left alone with young
   female children for a long period of time.   ( )

3. Sexual activity declines with age because of the loss
   of physical attractiveness of older men and women.   ( )

4. Sexual contact between an elderly woman and a
   young man is improper.   ( )

5. Unmarried people in nursing homes should not be
   permitted to have sex together, even if they request
   it.   ( )

6. Oral-genital sexual activity at any age shows an excessive desire for physical pleasure.   ( )

7. Elderly individuals should be encouraged to remain
   active sexually.   ( )

8. Only people who are married to each other should
   have sexual intercourse.   ( )

9. Premarital intercourse is much more common today than it was fifty years ago.   ( )

10. Masturbation is an acceptable way to experience
    sexual pleasure.   ( )

11. Sexual responsiveness is usually greater in women and men who have less education. ( )

12. Elderly couples should restrict their sexual activity to nighttime or to darkened rooms. ( )

13. Regular sexual functioning is important in later life for maintaining a sense of well-being. ( )

14. Married couples in nursing homes should have the freedom to engage in sexual intercourse, as long as it is in privacy. ( )

15. It is socially acceptable for an elderly unmarried man and an elderly unmarried woman to live together. ( )

16. Elderly persons with sexual problems should consult with their personal physician or a counselor. ( )

17. People remain sexual beings with needs and feelings throughout their lifetimes. ( )

2

Why Sex
in Later Life?

L ITTLE has been written about sexuality in later life. As a topic of scientific inquiry, late life sexuality has been studied only infrequently. In fact, until the past decade, the issue of sexuality in old age has virtually been ignored, even by gerontologists. This, of course, tells us something: sexuality in the aging is, at best, of marginal interest either to the professional gerontology community or to the public at large. Even older adults themselves have not shown much open interest in the topic, although they fill most workshops on late life sexuality whenever such workshops are offered.

The lack of interest in late life sexuality is a bit paradoxical, given American society's preoccupation with sex in general. A major magazine or newspaper tabloid would never leave the newsstands if it did not have a lead story with at least sexual innuendos. Popular television would probably fade away if it did not have sexual themes to build upon. So why the lack of interest in the sexuality of older people?

This benign neglect of late life sexuality may have many causes. We speculate that most of the causes result from the assumption that sexuality is not important to older people. We suspect that many people believe that the elderly simply outgrow their sexual needs. Conventional wisdom would argue that sexual interest will markedly decline with age and that sexual capacity will be severely compromised in an old body. There is, of course, some truth to both assumptions. Research does tell us that the physical intensity of the sex drive lessens somewhat with age and that chronic illness and general wear and tear on the body can modify sexual response. However, one should not assume that the meaning and significance of sexuality in the lives of older adults necessarily declines. The survey data on late life sexuality fully confirms the hypothesis that most elderly people continue to have sexual interests and feelings, and when health and opportunity permit, older adults remain or would like to remain sexually active.

As gerontologists, we must confess that our own appreciation of late life sexuality occurred unexpectedly. We had given little attention to the subject until we were asked to lecture on sexuality in the aging to the second-year medical students at our university. We had been asked to develop the lecture even though we were hardly professed experts on sexuality in the aged at that time. Fortunately, we had time enough both to review the literature and to sit down with some of our elderly friends and clients for help and insight. An eighty-six-year-old woman living in a nursing home gave us our first lesson on the significance of late life sexuality.

Our informant was a typical, small town woman who had been a wife, mother, and all-around citizen like thousands of others in her Midwest community. She was unexpectedly open and candid about her sexual life and pleased with our interest in her and her feelings. Sex had been an important and satisfying part of her young adult and adult life, and it remained so for her as an octogenarian. She told us that not only did she always enjoy sex, but, in her words, she "craved it." She remained sexually active well into her eighties, halted only by the death of her husband. To this day, she explained, she still had sexual thoughts and dreams. With a twinkle in her eye, she added, "But they are *only* dreams these days." She stated that throughout her life her sexual physiology always cooperated when she wanted sex, and she commented, "Even today, if I wanted sex, everything would work fine." Being in the nursing home depressed her because it was such a sexless environment. She felt that her coresidents "must be drugged or something. They are always sleeping." In parting from us, she reflected on her aging body and how she wished she could still be sexually active. We recorded this interview and have used it many times in our workshops.

Here we have a woman nearing the end of her life, well into her eighth decade, yet clearly very much a sexual human being. We probably would not find that all octogenarians feel as strongly as our informant did about sexuality, but that she did made us also reevaluate any assumptions we may have held about the meaning of sex for older persons.

Having become interested in the topic, we became formally involved in researching issues related to late life sexuality. Our area of interest has centered on the knowledge and attitudes of caregivers toward late life sexuality. Our studies revealed a level of ignorance that needed to be addressed, the foremost issue being the need to answer the question, "Why is sex important to older people?"

Out of our research, literature review, and many interviews with elders, we have developed what amounts to a philosophy of late life sexuality. This philosophy is our rationale for explaining the importance of teaching and learning about sexuality in the older adult.

Included in our philosophy of late life sexuality, is the awareness and acceptance of an older person's right to retire sexually (to cease having sexual intercourse). People retire sexually for many reasons, not all of them voluntary. When people do voluntarily retire sexually, it may be for a wide variety of reasons. As long as the choice is comfortable for the person and acceptable to his or her partner, sexual retirement will not necessarily compromise sexual health. Sexual health is so much more than simply sexual intercourse.

We are aware that each generation has been raised in a particular cultural environment. With the current generation of older persons, this generally has meant being raised in a somewhat restrictive sexual environment. Cultural and religious values tied sex more closely to procreation than to personal pleasuring. Before the general acceptability and availability of birth control, sexual intercourse meant the risk of pregnancy. Abortions were rarely if ever an acceptable alternative to an unwanted pregnancy. For those raised in such an environment, not surprisingly, sex could become threatening and less than satisfying to some people. In these cases, old age could provide a welcome reason to retire from unhappy sexual obligations (in marriage) or from unsatisfying sexual activity.

Sexual retirement may also occur because of sexual boredom with or general dislike of a partner. As love making becomes more a matter of routine than passion, its importance is assumed to diminish greatly, even to the point of sexual avoidance. The boredom theory, however, typically masks other problems, such as anger toward a sexual partner or historic discomfort with sexual activity itself. The fact that there is some routine to sex should not make it "boring," since for the most part we establish routines for quite opposite reasons. Having a routine allows one the satisfaction of the anticipation of the event, as well as the actual enjoyment of the event when it does take place. The mystery in sex may diminish over a lifetime, but the pleasure derived from the experience need not necessarily lessen. At any age, it is certainly possible and desirable to add some variety to love making to avoid boredom. However, if both partners enjoy sex and feel good about each other, the satisfaction is not in the physical technique or act but in the relationship itself.

Although we can understand and accept sexual retirement, sexual health probably is best maintained if and where a regular active sexual life is possible. The reasons for encouraging an active sexual life into old age (which constitute the basis of our philosophy regarding sex in later life) include the following:

Sex can act as an antidote to the idea of body as a repository of pain in old age

Sex can be a way of preventing social disengagement in old age

Sex can be a means for promoting and maintaining intergenerational understanding

Sex can be a safe and valuable form of physical exercise

Sex can be a way of maintaining a healthy self-image in old age

Sex can be a support in managing personal anxieties

Sex as an Antidote to Pain

As we age, we run the risk of developing chronic disease. Few of us will escape having one or more of these diseases, and our bodies will likely experience some measure of chronic pain, even while we receive careful medical management. Under such conditions, it is easy to start viewing our bodies as repositories of pain and only on rare occasions as capable of giving pleasure.

It seems that as we grow older, we pay more attention to food and drink, one of the more manageable ways in which we can experience pleasure through the body. The problem with food and drink is that, consumed beyond a certain point, they can be dangerous to our health. It is more than just the shifting of body weight with age that gives late middle-aged adults their girthy appearance. We suspect that many may have given up the bed for the table. Obviously, sex is one of the healthier ways in which we can counter some of the aches and pains that accompany aging. Knowing that we continue to have the capacity for sexual activity and the good feelings that it brings helps to reassure us that even a body that is no longer perfectly healthy is not really so bad.

Overcoming Social Disengagement

Although some gerontologists may have overstated the point, the observation that some older people "disengage" themselves from society as they get older has some truth to it. When mobility becomes limited and one's sensory equipment (particularly sight and hearing) is impaired, it is easy to retreat into oneself. We certainly know of a number of elderly people who essentially have withdrawn into themselves to await death.

How can one prevent such a pattern from developing? For most elderly, this will not be a problem. People who have lived their lives with vigor and enthusiasm usually continue to do so until death, despite all the things that can go wrong. Sexual activity, insofar as it usually requires a partner about whom one cares, is perhaps one of the best measures for preventing social disengagement. To cooperate in a sexual partnership generally means a willingness to invest energy and attention in the partner. It means sharing oneself with another person. How different this is from withdrawal behavior!

An Intergenerational Language

There is no denying the reality of intergenerational differences. The living family of humanity covers nearly a century. People born at different times, in different cultures, have different values and worldviews. This presents to young and old the challenge of finding ways to build intergenerational understanding and respect. The failure to understand one another can bring great pain to either group. When the young view the old as sexless, for example, great harm is done to both groups.

Recognizing that sexual interest and activity are a normal part of the life of an elderly person provides the basis of communication with the young, who typically are deeply involved in discovering their own sexual identities. Discovering that both young and old share the fears and the enjoyment that comes with sex should help each group better identify with the other. The young and the old need not be sex objects for one another for them to appreciate their respective sexual natures. The "dirty old man" idea got started because of a belief that old men somehow desired only young partners. This definitely is not true; research clearly shows that late life sexuality takes place between partners of relatively similar ages.

Sex as Exercise

Health and fitness are popular among people of all ages in the United States today. Never have so many taken up exercise in one form or another, such as walking, jogging, swimming, and aerobic dancing. Older adults are very much a part of this trend. The pursuit of fitness, however, is not without its dangers. Any form of exercise undertaken at an advanced age must be approached cautiously and employed judiciously. Injury or accidents are always possible.

Though we do not often think of it in these terms, sexual activity is a form of exercise. It is the aerobic equivalent of walking three blocks or climbing two and a half flights of stairs. Virtually all systems of the body are called upon in the completion of a sexual act. From the respiratory system to the neuromuscular system, the body is being exercised. But most important, the exercise is almost totally safe. In sexual activity there is no falling on slippery sidewalks or turning an ankle in an unseen pothole; such accidents do not occur if you are in bed. Sexual activity is a means to sexual health, which, in turn, is a contributor to total health.

A Positive Body Image

As we grow older, our bodies change, age. Such changes are given values by the culture in which we live. In our culture, an aging body is thought to lose beauty, not gain it. Wrinkles on the face, brown spots on the hands, and protruding veins in the legs are unwelcomed changes. They are also perceived as a sign of yet another loss, that of our physical attractiveness. If you add some pain because of disease to this picture of aging, you will understand why an older person may begin to experience some deterioration in the sense of self-image and even of self-worth. It is common for older people to be present but feel "unseen" as the eyes of others seem to avoid them. Since we cannot stop the aging process or, at least at the moment, redefine beauty for our culture, what can we do?

Sexual activity is based at least in part upon one's attractiveness to another person. We want to touch and embrace the loved or desired object of our affection and sexual stimulation. To be touched and embraced offers physical evidence that we are loved or desired. It means that whatever we are or whoever we are, it is more than enough to generate interest and physical response from a significant other. This relationship will certainly help to restore self-confidence and provide reassurance that an aging body has a beauty of its own and that the expression of sexual feelings is a communication between *people*, not bodies.

Coping with Challenges

At any age, life is challenging. Old age has its own sets of concerns. We worry about our health, whether we have enough retirement income, the possible loss of a spouse or loved one, the well-being of our adult children, and so on. Some people believe that old age is particularly heavy with anxiety-producing situations. Whether it is or not, the older person welcomes relief from such anxieties. We may go to the doctor, take pills, or seek out friends as part of this process. If we are fortunate to have still an interested partner, we can make love. At all ages, love making has been an outlet for defusing anxieties and for psychologically refueling ourselves to cope with life's challenges. The reassurance and energizing that come with a healthy love relationship, with or without the physical dimension, are a powerful medicine for facing the future.

We have described a number of benefits that late life sexuality may produce. As part of our philosophy of sexual health, we have avoided making sexual intercourse the centerpiece of late life sexuality and have recognized that sexual retirement may be an appropriate choice for some people. But when and where opportunity permits, the maintenance of a regular, active sexual life is definitely health promoting. It provides mental as well as physical benefits to the individual. Beyond this, a sexually active population of people over sixty helps remind others in our culture that growing old does not alter basic human needs, nor does it fundamentally change human capacities such as the ability to function sexually.

3

The Aging Body
and Physical Response

W E cannot deny the aging of our bodies. From middle age on, we bear witness to these changes every time we undress. A quick glance in the mirror reminds us of the origin of the expression, "the naked truth." The passing years are etched on our bodies as if on a daily diary.

It is unfortunate that our culture views the physical changes of middle and old age as negative ones. This perception often creates more problems for us sexually than do any changes in our sexual organs due to advancing years. The attitude that old bodies are ugly or not sexually interesting or enticing is an indictment of the shortsightedness of society. More than anything, it reflects a state of ignorance about the ongoing sexual nature of humankind. Thankfully, beauty remains in the eye of the beholder, and sexual turn-on is based in the mind of the beholder.

If we take a long look in our mirror, what do we find? Our gift wrapping (skin) sags and wrinkles according to our years, our hair thins and grays, added beauty spots appear, body weight likes to concentrate about our middles, and our arms and legs grow thinner. The strength and integrity of our muscles may be reduced, depending upon the regularity and extent of our exercise and daily activities. If we are inclined to explore the visible areas of our sexual anatomy, women will confess to sagging breasts and a protruding abdomen. Men will notice that the penis appears smaller, and the scrotal sac sags.

What we cannot see are the equally dramatic changes inside our bodies. Our central nervous system grows lazier, our circulatory system becomes slower and less efficient, and our endocrine system produces a different mix and volume of hormones. Since all these systems play a part in the efficiency of our sexual functioning, they combine to influence changes in our sexual functioning as older adults. The good news is that the combined internal and external changes in our bodies rarely inhibit successful sexual functioning, but these changes do, in fact, produce some changes in sexual response that need to be understood if we are to remain comfortable with and confident in our ongoing sexual activity as we age.

As we noted earlier, most adults who are interested in retaining full sexual capacity may do so. Researchers have confirmed that the majority of older adults choose to remain sexually active if health and opportunity permit. What we are less well able to document is the anxiety and uncertainty that older adults may experience in accommodating their aging bodies to continuing sexual interest and activities. The pain and frustration associated with this anxiety, however, often may be caused by simple ignorance. Few of us systematically learn about the aging process, let alone receive any form of adult sexual education. We simply muddle along, confused by our experiences and uncertain about whether our experiences are shared by our peers or are simply unique to ourselves. It would be easy to say "do what comes naturally" if only we knew what is natural at our age and circumstance in life. The bottom line (at all ages) is that we need to know and understand how the aging process affects sexual interest and capacity.

It is imperative that any differences in aging due to gender be understood and communicated between men and women who are sexual partners. Unfortunately, such partnerships in sexual activity are too often taken for granted. The subtle changes in sexual response may be easily overlooked, ignored, or misinterpreted. When this occurs, sexual dysfunction or failure may occur easily. To reduce anxiety, one of the sexual partners may choose to limit his or her sexual interest and even shelve future sexual activity. In effect, that partner sexually retires. When this happens, the sexual partnership may be severely or permanently damaged. If mutually acceptable to both partners, this may be of little consequence. However, where the decision is one-sided, it may cause irreparable damage to an otherwise healthy relationship. In view of the magnitude of such a decision, it is critical that we learn as much as science can offer about how age affects our ability to function as sexual beings.

Sex and the Older Man

Let us first explore what we know about the effects of aging on the sexual interest and activity of men. Men often identify their sexual anatomy with the penis. The penis is certainly a principal sexual organ of the male; however, it is not the only part of the male body involved in the male sexual response cycle. The testes, anal sphincter muscle, and even the breasts are involved in the sexual response of men. Changes in each of these parts of the male anatomy need to be explored. Thanks to the laboratory studies of Masters and Johnson (1986), we now have such intimate information; for a more detailed description of both male and female anatomy and of the physiology of sexual response, we refer our readers to their work.

Since the penis is assumed to be of such critical importance to male sexuality, let us see what happens to this organ in old age. Like any other muscular structure of the body, it loses some of its muscle tone and weight with age. As muscle tissue atrophies (shrinks), the penis inevitably will become smaller and less straight. Contrary to myth, the reduced size of the penis has little bearing on the sexual experience of one's partner during sexual intercourse. Sexuality as a partnership is usually complemented by the sexual anatomy of the female, whose vagina flexes to accommodate the size of the penis.

The penis of an older man is usually less hard than that of the younger at the point of erection. This is because the hardness results from the congestion of blood in the spongy tissues of the penis. Given the change in blood circulation throughout the body of the older male and the increased rigidity of the blood vessels with age, the congestion of blood will be slower and perhaps less effective. The result is both a longer period of time needed to achieve an erect penis, plus a somewhat softer penis at the point of erection. Generally, the penis of the healthy older man will be sufficiently hard to complete sexual intercourse, although it may not be able to penetrate the vagina of his sexual partner if intromission is attempted prematurely.

In those instances where the penis fails to harden sufficiently for intercourse because of physiological reasons, there are still several alternatives. Through a technique referred to as "stuffing," the partner may use her hands to ease and hold the penis in the vagina. Once entering has been accomplished, sexual excitement will usually facilitate hardening of the penis. In other situations, the male may be fitted with a penile prosthesis (implant), which allows the man to consummate intercourse. There are different kinds of penile implants, and the advantages and disadvantages of each need to be discussed with the physician. It is also important for both partners to realize that the erect penis produced by the implant will not be as long or as great in circumference as the patient's previous physiologic erections were, but in nearly all cases, those men who have had implants have been quite satisfied with the results (Benson 1985).

Once the penis is erect and the male has penetrated his partner, the man experiences an urgency for ejaculation. In the older male, this urgency is not as great as it is in most younger males and often is under greater voluntary control. This is a decided advantage for the older male, who can enjoy the period of sexual excitement far longer than can his younger counterparts, and this is often appreciated by his partner. In some older men, ejaculation may not occur with every instance of sexual intercourse, perhaps only every second or third time. The delay or nonoccurrence of ejaculation needs to be understood by both partners as quite normal; otherwise, it could be misconstrued as a form of impending impotency.

Ejaculation involves the contraction of the penis and the simultaneous expulsion of semen. This is the normal process for the male for releasing sexual tension created by sexual arousal and excitement. As men age, the intensity and frequency of these penile contractions lessen, and the force with which semen is expelled is reduced. In some instances in older men, this will be experienced as semen simply dripping off the end of the penis. Since both partners can sense the lessened intensity of this development, they need to be reassured that this is quite normal. Most important, both partners need to understand that this development has little bearing upon experiencing sexual interest or pleasure.

Orgasm in the male is experienced as the repeated contraction of the penis culminating in ejaculation. As has been noted, the intensity of this process decreases with age, causing the male orgasm to decrease in physical intensity. Generally, the number of penile contractions that occur is about half that of a younger male. How orgasm is experienced by an older man, however, may be as much or more a product of what is going on in his mind than any change in bodily function.

So far, we have discussed changes in the physical function of the penis and how it affects sexual performance. But the penis does not act alone in sexual intercourse. With sexual arousal, the nipples on the male breast become erect as sexual stimulation draws blood to the area. The blood congests to produce the nipple erection. In sexual excitement, the male testes elevate in the scrotal sac, and the muscles controlling the anal opening contract. In old age these associated physiological developments are slightly altered. The male nipple will become erect, but more slowly, because of the slower circulation of the blood and the looseness of the chest skin. The testes may not elevate at all, and the anal muscles may not contract as sharply. Again, none of these developments has any real bearing on the quality of the sexual experience.

Sex and the Older Woman

In the older woman (that is, postmenopausal), the changes in sexual anatomy are somewhat more dramatic. Given the intimate connection of the female anatomy to reproduction, cessation of the reproductive cycle (menopause) can be expected to have a significant impact on the female organs. The basis of these physical changes is the reduction of the female hormone estrogen. Estrogen is produced principally in the ovaries. When the ovaries cease to function, as they do with menopause, they shut down the production of this important hormone.

The loss of estrogen should not affect sexual interest in women, since sexual desire takes place in the head and the heart. However, the drop in estrogen has some direct bearing on the physical integrity of the vagina. The reduction of estrogen increases the thinning of the tissue walls of the vagina. The layers of this wall will decrease from eight layers to as few as four layers in the older woman. A thinned vaginal wall does not inhibit sexual performance, but it does increase the risk for certain complications when sexual intercourse occurs. Since the vaginal wall serves to cushion the urethra and bladder from the thrust and impact of the penis, the thinner wall allows greater potential shock and abrasion to these nearby organs. Irritation of the urethra and/or irritation of the bladder both can cause discomfort with sexual intercourse and must be treated immediately by a physician. Home remedies should not be attempted, for the delay in getting treatment may increase the severity of infection if bacteria are present.

Unfortunately, the thinning of the vaginal wall is not the only effect of a drop in estrogen levels. An equally disconcerting change is the reduced level of secretant that permeates the vagina in response to sexual excitement. With lower levels of this lubricant, sexual intercourse could be experienced as scratchy and may cause itching in the vagina. These symptoms can be alleviated by the use of personal lubricants, or in severe cases, estrogen creams or suppositories may be prescribed. If a personal lubricant is used, it is very important that it be a water-soluble product, such as K-Y Jelly; one may also choose to use a personal lubricant in suppository form. The use of petroleum-based products should be avoided, for such products may possibly harbor germs that can cause infection or produce an allergic reaction.

Estrogen is most important in maintaining the structure and physical integrity of the vagina. Length, width, and flexing ability all depend on suitable estrogen levels—and on regular sexual intercourse. Older women who have sexual intercourse only infrequently because of illness, loss of interest, or the loss of their partner can expect some shrinking of the vagina. Resumption of intercourse can cause some initial discomfort and should be anticipated in such cases. Knowledge of these changes needs to be understood and communicated by both partners. Given patience, the vagina will stretch and return to its ability to accommodate the penis. However, even with regular sexual activity, some shrinking and lack of muscle integrity will still occur in the vagina.

The outer lips of the vagina (the labia) will lose some of their muscle tone and will sag slightly. They will not hold the penis as tightly as they did in the past.

The female counterpart of the male penis is called the clitoris. It is located slightly above the opening of the vagina. This small, penislike organ is considered to be highly erogenous. Most women find gentle clitoral stimulation sexually arousing. In older women the clitoris retains its sexual sensitivity, but the fatty tissue cover, the hood that protects the clitoris, thins with age. Without this protective cover, this area may respond to insensitive touch by producing pain rather than pleasure. Aging sexual partners who are accustomed to using clitoral stimulation as part of sexual arousal need to pay particular attention to the tenderness of this organ. It is always preferable that couples openly discuss changes in their bodies' response to sexual activity.

Perhaps too much attention has been given to orgasm in the female. Popular literature has emphasized all the potential sexual highs that exist, given the right technique or technology. The older woman, however, can particularly suffer from this expectation, since her orgasmic experience will be altered with age. Like the older man, the older woman may misinterpret this change to mean that she is losing her sexual potency. Nothing could be further from the truth.

The female orgasm physiologically involves two concurrent body responses: the contractions of the wall of the vagina and the elevation of the uterus above the vagina. This occurs as a result of sexual stimulation. The woman's state of health, of course, is also important. In an older woman, because the vagina has undergone structural changes, it is less responsive, and its number of contractions (with orgasm) is reduced (to about half as many as in younger women). Also, with advanced age, the uterus will not elevate or will only partially elevate. Fortunately, these changes rarely diminish sexual satisfaction, although they do reduce the physical intensity of the orgasm. There are occasions, however, when the elevation of the uterus causes pain and diminishes the pleasure of orgasm; this may be related to lower levels of estrogen.

An important part of the female sexual anatomy is the breast. As in the male, the nipples of the female will become erect with sexual arousal. This occurs as the rush of blood triggered by sexual arousal congests in the area of the nipple. In older women, when the breasts droop and circulation slows, the nipple erection will be slowed, and the blushing (reddening of the skin) that occurs with the congestion of blood may be less evident. Other sexually sensitive parts of the female body may also lose some of their physical sensitivy due to the normal changes of aging. It is at this point that the mind (with its long history of memories of sexual experience) can help the body experience a full measure of pleasure. Interestingly enough, many of these physical changes that occur as a result of aging are absent or are much less severe in women who have regular sexual stimulation. This will be discussed more fully in chapter 7.

In summary, there is no denying growing old. We can feel it and see most of it. However, we remain sexual beings all of our lives, and for the most part, our sexual equipment can continue to function throughout the entire life cycle. What we lose in physical intensity, we make up for in the unhurried response to sexual arousal and in the pleasure of touch and contact without experiencing the premature urgency for intercourse. In old age, physical contact and stimulation may become more important than simply feeling the release of sexual tension with orgasm.

Since we are vulnerable to worrying about the loss of our sexual capacity, knowledge of how our bodies age sexually is critical. We need to know which changes are normal and which should be a reason for concern. Old age is also a period of increased illness and changes in health status. Any illness can affect sexual interest. Some illnesses and their treatment can affect the ability to function sexually. We will discuss some of these changes in the next chapter.

4

Chronic Illness and Sexuality

I T has been said that nobody dies of old age. Likewise, age alone is generally not responsible for sexual dysfunction in the later years. The advancing years may slow us down, but only disease and illness can provide a real roadblock to our sexual functioning. Along with widow- and widowerhood, physical illness presents the most challenging obstacle to remaining sexually healthy in later life. Regardless of how well we take care of ourselves, sooner or later we must face the arrival of chronic disease.

Any illness, acute or chronic, disturbs our sexual life, even when the illness does not directly affect the sexual organs themselves. Sexual response depends so heavily on the cooperation of all the systems of the body that trouble in any one of them (the hormonal, circulatory, or nervous systems) can disrupt our sexual functioning. In addition, because sexual response is so dependent upon our mental state, the highly distracting nature of illness tends to consume our energy in the attempt to restore health to our bodies. Thus, the psychic investment and energy needed for sexual interest and response are depleted. Nearly any disease can be a culprit in cheating us of our libido. However, for the purposes of this chapter, we will limit our discussion to the impact of some of the more common chronic illnesses on sexual functioning.

Coping with Heart Disease

Heart disease remains one of the most common chronic diseases experienced in later life. Nearly one in three older persons can expect to experience some form of heart trouble. Heart disease takes many forms, ranging from hypertension (high blood pressure) to myocardial infarcts (heart attacks) to cerebral vascular accidents (strokes). Each of these disease entities presents its own challenge to sexual functioning.

Hypertension, fortunately, is relatively easy to control. When high blood pressure is adequately controlled, the likelihood of coronary artery disease, heart attacks, or stroke is lessened. As a disease, hypertension does not pose any great threat to sexual life. Sexual activity may elevate blood pressure slightly and accelerate the heart and respiratory (breathing) rates, but not enough to contribute to a heart attack. The physical demands of sexual intercourse are relatively minimal, requiring about the same amount of physical energy as climbing twenty steps (Renshaw 1981) or walking briskly for a few blocks. When sexual function is affected by hypertension, the problem is most likely to be caused by the medications used to treat the disease, rather than by the disease itself. These medications will be discussed in the next chapter.

After an older person has experienced a heart attack, the medical routine usually includes the limitation of physical exertion, including cessation of sexual activity. The damaged heart muscle requires time, without any undue stress, to heal. However, following this initial healing period, patients are allowed to increase gradually their physical exercise in one form or another. It has been customary to advise patients to wait eight to fourteen weeks before resuming normal sexual activities with a familiar partner. Butler and Lewis (1976) suggest that masturbation can be resumed earlier than this, and at least one recent researcher believes that sexual intercourse can be resumed at one month after a heart attack (Benson 1985).

To the person who has suffered a heart attack, having a damaged or injured heart may be very distressing emotionally. Fear and anxiety often accompany the decision to resume the activities of daily living, which include the resumption of sexual activity. What is feared, of course, is another heart attack. The wise physician and the considerate sexual partner may both be needed to help the heart patient return to sexual health. The physician can reassure the patient that the physical demands of sexual activity are less than most other routines of daily living, and that subsequent heart attacks due to stress from sexual intercourse virtually never occur. When heart attacks have occurred during sexual intercourse, they have almost always been caused by the patient's having sex with a new partner, with a younger partner (an older man/younger woman combination), or in unfamiliar circumstances. In other words, the underlying factor was not the physical demands of sexual intercourse, but the psychic stress produced by the guilt or excitement associated with the particular choice of place or partner. Other reported cases have shown that heart attacks during sexual activity occurred after a heavy meal or excessive alcohol consumption.

For many years, doctors have commonly recommended reducing physical stress in sexual relations for heart patients by suggesting a change in position for sexual intercourse. It was assumed that if a male heart attack patient took the bottom position during intercourse, then the risk of precipitating another heart attack or producing chest pain due to exertion would be reduced. Recent research, however, has demonstrated that the actual position in intercourse has little effect on the physical energy demanded by the body. If chest pain (angina pectoris) occurs during sexual intercourse, nitroglycerin or a similar medication is usually recommended (Scheingold and Wagner 1974).

The considerate sexual partner is important because the cessation of sexual activity for an eight-to-fourteen-week period may produce some physical changes in the sexual anatomy, especially for women, that could present some problems. For the older woman, the absence of sexual activity for this long a period can result in some shrinking, narrowing, and rigidity of the walls of the vagina. The attempt to resume sexual intercourse may be accompanied by pain until the vagina regains some of its physical integrity through the resumption of sexual activity. It is also important for both partners to realize that if it is the male partner who is recovering from a heart attack, any anxiety or apprehension about resuming sexual activity may precipitate an episode of temporary impotence (inability to have an erection).

If several such episodes take place, they should be discussed with a sympathetic physician or counselor to prevent permanent impotence.

One danger of involuntary sexual retirement that occurs because of serious illness is that the illness may present an excuse for not resuming sexual activity. If both partners had been looking for a face-saving way to retire sexually and the decision to do so is mutually agreeable, then perhaps there is no issue. However, if one partner uses the heart attack as an excuse to retire sexually against the wishes of the other, a definite strain in the relationship may occur. That is why it is very important for health care personnel who are following a heart patient to take a sexual history and to maintain an open counseling relationship with the patient and the sexual partner.

Unlike the heart attack, the cerebral vascular accident (stroke) poses no direct threat to the physiology of the sexual response (Gupta and Singh 1981). No damage to the heart results from a stroke, although other parts of the body may be affected with paralysis or limited function as a consequence of the stroke, depending upon the part of the brain affected by the stroke. Nonetheless, a stroke can affect sexual function. The effects, however, are indirect and are primarily mental (Bray et al. 1981).

Common emotional responses to stroke include depression and frequent mood swings, which may alternate between inappropriate crying and laughing. These feelings, coupled with the sense of losing attractiveness because of residual paralysis or speech impediments, can rob one of needed sexual energy. A stroke often causes greater injury to the spirits than to the body. In the eyes of our sexual partner, especially a long-term sexual partner, we may have changed little. In our own eyes, however, we may feel violated and fear that we are no longer sexually interesting or inviting. In such cases, time and tender, loving support can and should permit a return to reasonably full sexual activity. Severe or residual paralysis may complicate the ease with which we can respond sexually, and changes in the positions used for sexual intercourse may be necessary. Some of the alternate positions described in the section on arthritis in this chapter may be considered. But remaining sexually active will in no way precipitate another stroke.

Cancer and the Older Adult

This dreaded disease may develop in almost any area of the body, including areas of our sexual anatomy. Penile and prostate cancer in men, and breast and cervical cancer in women are obviously disruptive to sexual activity. Cancers in other areas of the body, depending upon the severity and the course of treatment required, may affect sexual interest and desire without necessarily affecting sexual physiology or performance. Cancers that require surgery or radical therapies may produce some disfigurement. As with stroke, if such disfigurement is perceived as a loss of personal attractiveness, it may disrupt normal sexual responsiveness.

Given the early detection and improved treatment of many forms of cancer, the gains in life expectancy following treatment mean that sexual retirement is no longer inevitable. It does become a time, however, when love and intimacy are needed more than ever. Sexual and intimate expression can contribute to making each day count for the cancer patient, even for those who are clearly terminally ill.

Questions regarding sexuality, emotional counseling, and any other aspects of cancer and its treatment may be directed to trained staff members of the National Cancer Institute by calling the Cancer Information Service (CIS). The toll-free telephone number is 1-800-4-CANCER. All calls are confidential. There is an excellent free booklet, *Advanced Cancer: Living Each Day*, which is available from the Office of Cancer Communications, National Cancer Institute, Building 31, Room 10A18, Bethesda, MD 20205. In addition to a great deal of practical information, the booklet contains a listing of organizations and resources for cancer patients, families, and caretakers.

Much has been written about cancers of the breast and uterus in women and about the significance of their removal. There is a common belief that such surgeries must inevitably interfere with sexual responsiveness in women who undergo these operations (Butler and Lewis 1976). However, research shows that neither surgery disrupts the physiology of sexual response. There may be a loss of sexual interest, desire, or even orgasmic response, but this is an affair of the mind, not the body.

Efforts are constantly being made to reduce the negative side effects of cancer therapy, and cancer patients may find themselves feeling well enough to maintain a reasonably active sexual life, or at least to be able to look forward to a return to satisfying sexual expression once the treatments are completed.

Prostatitis and Impotence

Prostate disease is common among older males. Nearly one-third of the male population over age sixty-five will experience some form of prostate disease, the most common being the enlarged prostate, which can interfere with bladder function. Prostatitis is characterized by a cloudy white discharge from the penis. Some pain in the area between the scrotum and anus and in the end of the penis on urination may be experienced. The presence of pain in this sensitive area may diminish sexual desire, especially if pain is experienced with ejaculation.

Most prostate problems are treatable. External treatment (warm baths and gentle massage) may be all that is needed. Surgical procedures, however, are common, and most will relieve the pain; following convalescence, most patients will be able to resume sexual activity comfortably. The most severe form of prostate surgery, the perineal procedure (which is discussed more fully in the next chapter), may produce irreversible impotence. In these cases, patients will be advised to pursue alternate avenues of sexual pleasure or consider a penile prosthesis.

A booklet, *Impotence After Cancer Surgery*, may be requested from the Impotence Information Center, American Medical Systems, P.O. Box 9, Minneapolis, MN 55440. This publication discusses impotence that occurs after cancer surgery involving the prostate, bladder, colon, and rectum. Many major insurance companies (check your own company specifically) and Medicare will provide benefits for penile implant surgery when impotence is caused by an organic or physical problem.

Although some people still believe that impotence is primarily a psychological problem, a growing number of professionals believe that as many as 75 percent of cases may have organic causes, either disease or the drugs used to treat the disease (Spark, White, and Connolly 1980). We urge men suffering from impotence to seek consultation from a specialist (usually a urologist) before accepting a diagnosis of irreversible impotence.

Arthritis

Perhaps the chronic disease most frequently complained about by the older adult is arthritis. There are really several forms of this disease: osteoarthritis and rheumatoid arthritis and related disorders. In older persons, more than one form of arthritis is often present simultaneously. Osteoarthritis is the pain and stiffness associated with the wear and tear on our bone structure. We become most aware of this disease when we observe some disfigurement in our fingers and legs. The changes of osteoarthritis are visible in the curvature (bowing) of these digits and limbs. Apart from the disfigurement, there is really no systemic disease process operating that could impair sexual function in any way, but the stiffness and pain in various joints may make some positions for sexual intercourse uncomfortable, depending upon the joints involved.

Rheumatoid arthritis is one of a group of systemic diseases that affects the joints, muscles, and tendons, and produces pain that seems to endure for long periods. Because of the discomfort produced by movement, persons with low pain thresholds often reduce activity and movement in an effort to avoid pain. Unfortunately, this only causes the joints to "freeze up" from disuse and increases the pain and discomfort, if and when movement of the joints is necessary.

Included in the rheumatic diseases are two other disorders that may cause difficulties with sexual activity: Sjogren's syndrome and scleroderma. Both of these conditions affect the mobility of the joints and muscles. Women with either of these disorders will frequently experience a marked lack of vaginal lubrication beyond that which characterizes normal aging, and they will need to use a water-soluble personal lubricant during intercourse (Arthritis Foundation 1985; United Scleroderma Foundation 1983). Men with scleroderma may also experience a condition called Peyronie's disease, which causes a painful erection that may make intercourse impossible at times. Although this condition is usually described as rare, Butler and Lewis (1976) believe that it occurs more often than was originally thought. Various treatments are available, and a urologist should be consulted.

Obviously, sexual activity requires considerable range and motion of the limbs and joints. There is a small measure of athleticism in having sexual intercourse. It is very important that sexual partners communicate openly about which sexual activities and expressions of intimacy are pleasurable and which may produce pain. At times the person with any form of arthritis or the other rheumatic diseases may find even a simple embrace painful, and the sexual partner may become afraid to hug or caress because of the fear of causing pain. Some of the medications used to control pain may also affect sexual desire and performance.

The arthritic person needs to keep in mind that the sore joint is not harmed but helped by use and exercise. Sexual intercourse is one of the most pleasurable physical activities, and as a by-product it helps to maintain some range and motion of the joints and limbs, as well as possibly to stimulate the body's production of cortisone, which is one of the substances used to treat the symptoms of rheumatoid arthritis (Cochrane 1984).

Therapy for arthritis usually includes medication to control pain and the recommendation that patients exercise to keep the joints functioning. Pain during sexual intercourse may also be minimized by experimenting with alternative positions. Examples of these are provided on pages 40–41 in figures 4–1 through 4–7, which have been reproduced from the Arthritis Foundation publication, *Living and Loving: Information About Sex* (Arthritis Foundation, 1982).

A warm bath, massage of painful joints, and timing the use of analgesics (pain-killing medication) approximately thirty minutes prior to intercourse may also help to control some of the pain associated with arthritis. Some patients with rheumatoid arthritis find that sexual activity is most enjoyable in the morning when they are well rested; others find that there is too much stiffness in the joints at this time. Again, communication between partners is essential. Some people find that using a satin sheet as the bottom sheet on the bed helps mobility. In addition, an inflatable pillow ("Compata-Pillow") can be placed under the woman's hips to make intercourse more comfortable. This product and other health aids particularly designed for people with arthritis may be found in various home health catalogues (see appendix B). Sears stores are one readily available source. In many communities there are self-help groups for those who suffer from arthritis. Members of these groups often share helpful suggestions for making the tasks of daily living less stressful and painful, and they often share information concerning new products that have proved helpful in coping with their disease.

Treating Diabetes

Although not a disease exclusive to the elderly, diabetes is a common chronic ailment in many older adults. Only a small percentage of older adults have early onset or juvenile diabetes. This is fortunate, since older men who have been diabetic a good part of their lives may face eventual impotence. The impotence occurs because the disease interferes with the circulatory and neurologic mechanisms responsible for the supply of blood flowing to the penis for erection. Such men may be candidates for a penile implant. This possibility should be discussed by both partners and the health care professional.

The late onset diabetic male may experience some difficulties in establishing an erection, especially in the prediagnostic stage of the illness when the disease is still untreated (Ellenberg 1980). One of the diagnostic clues of diabetes in males is, in fact, impotence. Problems associated with erectile failures often lead the older man into believing that *age* may be the culprit and can cause him to delay seeking treatment. Once the diabetes is under control, potency usually returns.

In comparative studies of the effects of diabetes on sexual functioning, women diabetics are relatively unimpaired, although it is harder to document problems in women because they do not have a readily observable response comparable to erection (Ellenberg 1980). Diabetes may, however, weaken the sexual drive like any other major disease, simply out of preoccupation with one's state of health and feelings of personal well-being.

Diabetes, as a chronic disease, cannot be cured in the strict sense, but it can be controlled. The approaches to containing and managing

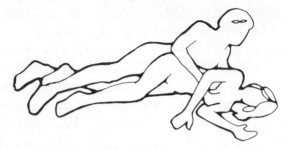

Figure 4–1. Both partners are lying on their side. The man enters from behind. The woman can have a pillow between her knees. This position is good if the woman has hip involvement.

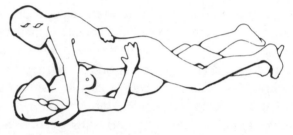

Figure 4–2. The woman lies on her back, knees together, with a pillow under her hips and thighs. Notice that the male partner is supporting his own body weight on his hands and knees. This position can be used when the woman has hip or knee involvement, or is unable to move her legs apart.

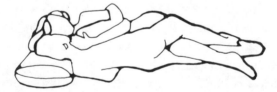

Figure 4–3. Side position with the partners facing each other. This can be used if the man has back involvement. Notice that in the positions described in figures 4–3 and 4–7 the woman must provide most of the hip movement.

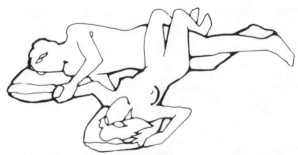

Figure 4–4. The woman lies on her back with her knees flexed. This position can be used when the woman has severe contractures.

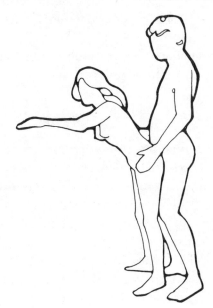

Figure 4–5. Both partners are standing. The man enters from behind. The woman uses furniture at a comfortable height for support and balance.

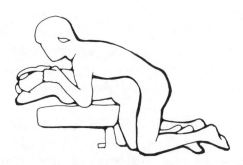

Figure 4–6. The woman is kneeling, her upper body supported by furniture. Her knees can be supported by a pillow. This position may be helpful if the woman has hip problems. Not good if the shoulders are involved.

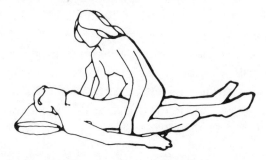

Figure 4–7. The man lies on his back. He may use pillows for support. The woman can support her own body weight on her elbows and/or knees. This position can be used when the man has hip or knee involvement.

the illness are directed toward changes in diet and through insulin replacement where appropriate. Once the blood chemistry is balanced and maintained, sexual problems attributable to the disease should disappear or become less severe.

Organic Brain Disorders

Organic brain disorders are among the most feared chronic illnesses experienced by older adults. This is particularly evidenced by the public attention focused on Alzheimer's disease. Alzheimer's disease is only one of many types of organic brain disease, but because of its progressive nature and the shortened life expectancy it causes, it remains the most feared.

The actual cause of Alzheimer's disease has not been established, although research into the general area of dementia shows a wide variety of conditions that may produce the symptoms of dementia: confusion, impaired thinking, dulled emotions, restlessness and irritability, even delusions and hallucinations.

Anemia, chemical addictions, subclinical infections, subclinical strokes, brain tumors, and depression may produce classical symptoms of dementia. Where organic brain damage is present, true dementia is seen; where such damage has not occurred, the problem is called pseudodementia.

There is no demonstrable evidence that real dementia necessarily produces a loss of interest in or a decreased capacity for sexual function. In fact, the mythology surrounding this disease suggests that hypersexual activity may actually occur as a result of impairment in social judgment. In its mild forms, the dependency that organic brain disease creates in its victims may result in more attentive and solicitous care by a spouse or significant other. Routine sexual patterns should suffer no major disruptions among couples in which one or both suffers from mild dementia. However, in the more severe form of dementia, the irrational behavior of the victim can be disruptive to close relationships with caring individuals. Angry outbursts, irritability, and paranoia damage the sexual attractiveness of the victims and reduce the sexual interests of their partners.

Overcoming Nutritional Disorders

Nutritional anemias are common in older persons, particularly among elderly women, and are the result of a reduction in the number or size of red blood cells or in the amount of hemoglobin the red blood cells contain. The most common form of anemia is caused by a deficiency of iron, but anemias can result from a deficiency of protein, vitamins, or other trace elements. This disorder usually originates in poor dietary habits; it can also result from poor absorption of nutrients because of other diseases or medications, or simply because our bodies may absorb nutrients less efficiently as we age. Many different explanations have been given for poor diets among older women, especially those who live alone. In some cases it comes down to not having enough money to purchase the variety of meats and fresh fruits and vegetables needed for a proper diet. Lack of appetite due to depression or to failure to eat properly because of physical or mental impairment may also be the basis for the anemia. The anemia, in turn, may contribute to further depression and to a lack of energy. Whatever the cause, nearly one in four elderly women suffers from anemia, and the condition is known to reduce sexual interest and desire (Butler and Lewis 1976). Again, it is not uncommon for a man or woman to attribute a loss or a marked reduction of sexual interest and desire to aging rather than to the real culprit—a treatable or manageable disease they may be experiencing. Fortunately, nutritionally caused anemias are easy to detect on laboratory examination and are also remediable with proper diet and iron or other nutritional supplements. However, it is important to follow the advice of a physician in treating anemias of any kind, rather than attempting self-treatment.

Anemia is just one of a number of dietary-related problems that have antiaphrodisiac effects. Equally common are the problems of overeating and the obesity that may result as they relate to sexual interest. This is not meant to imply that overweight men or women necessarily are sexually less attractive because of their size. However, excessive food intake may serve as a substitute for sexual expression in some older people. Food is used for oral pleasure, and the psyche is soothed by the awareness of "being fed." For some older adults, food has the advantage of not necessarily requiring a partner and not exposing one to the failure that could occur in a sexual encounter.

What is true of excessive food intake is even more true of excessive alcohol consumption. Alcoholism is believed to be a common chronic illness of older adults. For the male who has been a heavy drinker for a long time, the cumulative effects of alcoholism may result in impotence. Likewise, for the late onset heavy drinker, the toxic effects or sedative effects of the alcohol can make sexual function more difficult. The irony of alcohol use is that while it may arouse the sexual appetite, it does not help the follow-through. After a few alcohol-induced sexual failures, the older man will be inclined to give up and, sadly, in some cases, drink even more.

Many people have discussed the idea of alcohol as an aphrodisiac— something that makes one feel sexy. There is some truth to this. A mild amount of alcohol may loosen inhibitions and release some sexual energy. Beyond its very moderate use, however, alcohol has nothing but a deleterious effect on sexual health.

Fortunately, in many instances, reduction in the abuse level of alcohol through treatment or voluntary self-control can restore at least some of the lost sexual function. This will be most evident in the case of the older male with the restoration of penile erection.

Smoking is often associated with alcohol use (although there certainly are smokers who do not use alcohol). Smoking is yet another oral habit that introduces a toxic chemical into the body—nicotine. Nicotine is not only habit forming—that is, one can develop a true addiction to the substance—but it has also been known to cause impotence in men (Smith and Talbert 1986). For persons with chronic lung disorders, smoking only contributes to further impairment of lung function. Sexual dysfunction has been known to worsen as lung disease progresses, and chronic obstructive pulmonary disease may be associated with male impotence (Fletcher and Martin 1982).

Dealing with Low Back Pain

Another chronic disorder that plagues older adults and that can interfere with sexual activity is lower back pain. Since older persons often develop sedentary life patterns, sudden use of the back muscles can precipitate the problem. This is perhaps most likely to happen to men who are asked or expected to be the "lifters" in society. For women the circumstances are different. In the postmenopausal woman, the loss of estrogen (the female hormone) fosters osteoporosis or thinning of the bone structure, which can make bones and joints fragile and subject to fracture. The softer spine can also lead to lower back pain in women. In either case, the tissue that separates and cushions the spinal discs from each other often atrophies (shrinks) with age. When the tissue is so reduced that bone touches bone, back discomfort will occur. Osteoporosis is more easily prevented at an earlier age (by adequate calcium intake and regular exercise) than treated when one is older, but women with osteoporosis should follow their physician's advice regarding measures to prevent worsening of their condition as they age.

For chronic low back pain, little reversible repair is possible, although back surgery is possible in some cases. Usually people with the problem are assisted in finding ways to minimize their discomfort—by using firm mattresses or plywood boards between the mattress and bed springs, for example. The other form of treatment is exercise, especially for those with slipped discs or arthritic backs. Here sexual activity may serve as an excellent form of exercise for the back, stomach, and pelvic muscles. If lower back pain is a problem during sexual intercourse, some change in positioning may relieve or reduce the pain. For example, one such change is for the person with the back pain to assume the bottom position in sexual intercourse or for both partners to assume a side-by-side position. Some of the positions described earlier in this chapter may be helpful in relieving stress on the lower back in one or both partners.

This chapter covers some of the most common chronic physical illnesses and how they may or may not interfere with sexual interest and function in older adults. This discussion is by no means exhaustive but is intended to emphasize that illness does not signal the end of sexual expression for either the partner who is experiencing the onset of an acute or chronic illness or for the sexual partner. It is also intended to stress the need for older adults and those who care for them to recognize, anticipate, and discuss sexual concerns.

Sexual health is best served by maintaining good physical health, and sexual activity is believed to have a positive therapeutic value in maintaining good health in general. Obviously, the two are closely associated.

5

Medical Treatment— Implications for Sexuality

W E have just described some of the ways in which illness can produce serious impediments to our sexual health. Ironically, the treatment of an illness also can challenge our sexual vigor and, in fact, can give credence to the expression, "the cure is worse than the disease."

The treatment of an acute or chronic illness can take many forms. In our culture, medical practitioners commonly rely heavily on medications and surgeries to take care of what ails us. In the case of the various cancers, additional therapies such as radiation and chemotherapy may be employed, and in the case of kidney disease, dialysis may be used. In the best of circumstances, medical practitioners will back up such interventions with counsel and education. In other instances, we may have to seek counseling on our own and educate ourselves about the possible effects of a particular illness and about the implications of a proposed treatment for ourselves and our sexual partners.

This chapter will briefly explore how drugs, surgery, and other therapies may be associated with changes in our interests and ability to function sexually. Of necessity, the information will be quite general. In the most serious illnesses (for example, cancer), treatment may be highly individualized, and we can only strongly encourage the individual and his or her sexual partner to seek counseling and to discuss openly sexual concerns as they relate to their particular situation. Many of the more serious illnesses that affect older adults require highly sophisticated therapies that usually are found only in major medical centers, such as university-affiliated teaching hospitals. Patient education materials and counseling are more commonly available at these centers, and you may want to inquire about the availability of this information. Throughout the chapter, we frequently recommend the use of self-help groups where they exist, and we have included suggestions for easily obtainable booklets where they are available.

The Effect of Drugs

The older adult is increasingly at risk for a major illness, particularly one or more of the so-called chronic illnesses (for instance, hypertension, arthritis, and diabetes). In such chronic illnesses, the treatment may also be "chronic"—enduring, in other words. An adult with chronic hypertension (high blood pressure), for example, will be expected to take a prescribed medication for the duration of his or her life. These medications can have both immediate side effects and long-term side effects as the *toxic* damage created by a drug accumulates over time. Whether the effects are immediate or long-term, some medications may alter one's sexual drive and/or the responsiveness of one's sexual equipment. A sobering statistic is that people over age sixty represent 14 percent of the population but consume 30 percent of the prescribed drugs (Butler and Lewis 1976). Few older persons will remain free of a prescribed medication for any length of time.

Sexual function is dependent upon the good working order and collaboration of a number of systems in the body (that is, the nervous system, the circulatory system, the hormonal system, and so forth). Drugs that inhibit or otherwise alter the performance of any one of these systems could have the side effect of altering sexual response. For example, consider a medication that would "slow" blood flow through the body. The male penis depends upon blood flow for erection. A medication that slows the movement of blood could have the unintended effect of delaying erection or permitting only a partial erection, and this could be a very frustrating experience for the unsuspecting victim. For both men and women, sexual activity of any kind requires the presence of a drive or urge for sexual expression. Some medications may inhibit or reduce sexual drive; others, such as L-dopa, which is used in the treatment of Parkinson's disease, have been reported to increase temporarily the sexual drive in some patients, which may be disconcerting to the patient or the sexual partner.

Implicating any particular medication in an altered sexual responsiveness is difficult. We all respond to medication in our own ways; a drug that depresses sexual responsiveness in one person may have no effect on another. If we are taking more than one medication, a drug interaction may be responsible. Each drug alone may not produce any problems, but the combination may do so. As we grow older, the increase in the proportion of fat in the body means that some drugs remain in the tissues longer, and we may require lower doses of a drug than do younger persons. It is also important to remember that over-the-counter drugs that can be purchased without a prescription (for that reason, we often consider them to be harmless) may also interact with prescribed medications.

Our minds as well as our bodies can contribute to altered sexual response. The anxiety produced by an illness or by the need for medication may be as important as the medication itself in changing our sexual responsiveness or functioning.

For the person who questions whether a given medication may be responsible for a lack of sexual interest or for the inability to respond to sexual stimulation, we recommend looking up the stated side effects of the medication in the *Physicians' Desk Reference* (Medical Economics 1986). This reference should be available in your local library, or you may ask your pharmacist or physician to share this information with you. Over-the-counter drugs may be looked up in *Self-Medication: A Guide to Over-the-Counter Health Care Products* (Medical Economics Company 1984). In addition, a frank discussion with your personal physician or pharmacist might be helpful. You cannot automatically assume that your health practitioner will inform you of all the possible side effects of a medication, particularly those related to sexual function. In some cases, this may be due to the practitioner's assumption that an elderly patient is sexually inactive. In other cases, the practitioner may fear that the suggestion of a side effect will, in fact, cause the patient to experience it. In any case, we believe that it is imperative for elderly patients (and all patients, for that matter) to report any changes in sexual function that appear to be related to their medication. These patients may be able to take another medication that will treat the illess without affecting sexual function. It is very important to have a health practitioner with whom you feel comfortable discussing these matters; if you do not have such a health professional, perhaps you should look for one who is informed about and sympathetic to the sexual concerns of the older patient. As the availability of professionals trained in geriatrics increases, finding such help will become an easier task.

As we have mentioned, nearly any drug may affect sexual functioning in a given individual. However, several classes of prescription drugs are commonly reported to have an effect on sexual function in older adults. Antihypertensive medications, which are used to treat high blood pressure, and drugs used to treat psychiatric illnesses (antipsychotics, tranquilizers, and antidepressants) are the most commonly reported groups of drugs that may adversely affect sexual functioning, particularly in men (Curb et al. 1985; Smith and Talbert, 1986). These drugs may also affect sexual functioning in women, but the changes are more difficult to document because women do not have a sexual response as readily observable as do men (erection). The most frequent sexual problems reported by men who are treated with either of these classes of drugs include impotence (the inability to have or sustain an erection), decreased sexual drive, delayed ejaculation or an inability to ejaculate, enlargement of the breasts, and priapism (prolonged, painful erection). Women have reported problems with decreased vaginal lubrication, decreased sexual drive, and a delay or inability to achieve orgasm. A recent report in a popular magazine (*Better Homes and Gardens Health Update* 1986) offers a ray of hope in regard to the side effects of blood pressure medications. A new class of drugs called ACE inhibitors has been reported to cause fewer of the side effects that have caused patients to stop taking their blood pressure medication. Not all individuals are able to take these drugs, but it certainly warrants checking with a physician if your current medication is causing problems. We would also caution those who have discontinued using their blood pressure medication because of its effect on sexual function to be persistent in trying other medications. The danger of more serious heart disease or stroke from uncontrolled blood pressure is very high, and researchers have found that untreated high blood pressure also has harmful consequences for sexual function (Smith and Talbert 1986).

The drugs used in various chemotherapy regimens for the treatment of cancers affect sexual function in both men and women, and will be discussed later in this chapter. It is important to note that the use of drugs reported to have an aphrodisiac and/or mood-altering effect (for example, marijuana) may actually have the opposite effect on both sexual interest and function when used in high doses or for long periods of time (Burkhalter 1978).

Unfortunately, this description of potentially problematic drugs is not complete. New drugs are placed on the market every day. Some have had only limited studies of their effects on older adults; even less attention may have been paid to unintended effects on sexual functioning, particularly in men. Again, it is important to stress the need to report any observed change in sexual function that occurs after taking a newly prescribed medication.

The groups of drugs discussed here are used to treat a variety of conditions in which prescribed medications may have sexual consequences. Included are such problems as high blood pressure and other heart disorders, mental illness (including depression), and cancers. You will note that these are conditions in which the illness itself also may alter sexual response. Thus both the illness and the treatment may combine to disrupt sexual desire and response.

This presents us with a real dilemma. How important is our general health in relation to our sexual health? The decision should be ours, yet it is rarely considered when we consult with our health care professionals. This is not meant to imply a distrust of those who care for us, or that we advocate ignoring the advice of those to whom we entrust our health care. We simply wish to underscore the importance of exploring all the options available when reconciling the desire for active sexual expression with the potential side effects of proposed therapies.

Not all drugs, of course, are prescribed by health professionals, as we mentioned when discussing those purchased over the counter. A wide variety of over-the-counter (OTC) drugs are self-prescribed and used heavily by older adults for many problems. Unfortunately, alcohol also is consumed heavily by some older adults. Both OTC drugs and alcohol can alter sexual response. As they are absorbed into the body, they can inhibit the functioning of other bodily systems required for sexual performance. Given the vast array of OTC drugs available, it is difficult to point out any particular one as the source of the problem. However, in the case of alcohol, there is no equivocation, and one should remember that in combination with some drugs, alcohol is likely to increase the potential for dangerous side effects. It is imperative that you inquire about the possibility of such side effects if you are taking drugs and consuming alcohol, even if it is only a small quantity of the latter.

Alcohol is definitely a "downer." A little alcohol may light us up sexually (increase libido); more than a little has the opposite effect. Sexual desire may remain, but sexual performance is inhibited. Alcohol typically makes the consumer drowsy and unresponsive, a condition that does not lend itself to sexual activity.

We know that as we age, our bodies become less efficient at removing toxic chemicals from the bloodstream. Whether it is a prescribed medication or alcohol, a little goes a long way in an aging body. Someone who was accustomed to drinking heavily when younger may discover that even drinking a smaller amount will produce negative consequences for sexual function in later adulthood. Fortunately, alcoholism is treatable, and our consultants tell us that the recovery rates are even better for older adults than for younger persons. In many communities, both Alcoholics Anonymous and community mental health centers often provide special groups for older adults with alcohol-related problems, as well as counseling for partners and other family members. If you are the partner or relative of someone for whom alcohol is a problem, you may have to exert considerable pressure to cause the victim to seek treatment. Most individuals who suffer from alcohol dependence are "sincerely deluded," and they do not believe that they have a problem, even though it is obvious to everyone else (Haugland 1985).

Needless to say, what is true of alcohol is equally true of the heavy use of the so-called recreational drugs (marijuana, cocaine, heroin, or their synthetic substitutes). In effect, the artificial kick of these drugs overshadows natural sexual pleasure. It bears emphasizing that such drugs usually cause damage to our bodies, while sexual pleasure, for the most part, is health giving.

A Better Diet

Food intake (our diet) can have an impact on sexual function. As food is absorbed, it becomes part of our blood chemistry. Moderate and balanced eating enhances our bodily systems. Immoderate eating and unbalanced diets upset these systems. In so doing, sexual response may be disrupted. As we mentioned earlier (chapter 3), the circulatory system frequently becomes less efficient with age. Although the sharing of a meal may be a romantic prelude to making love, we recommend that the meal be a light one, for the diversion of blood flow required to digest a large, heavy meal may actually interfere with sexual functioning in an older adult.

We noted earlier that anemia, particularly in women, has been linked with a decrease in sexual libido. Overeating can act like a recreational drug—the pleasure that comes with eating may overshadow one's interest in sexual pleasure. A moderate and balanced food intake contributes both to general health and sexual health in later life.

Surgery

A major form of medical treatment is surgery. Even minor surgery may be distracting for an older person and may require an extended period of convalescence. Surgeries that involve areas associated with our sexual anatomy are definitely troublesome to our sexual health.

For example, one out of every three men over age sixty-five will experience prostate difficulties, usually inflammation or enlargement of the prostate gland. Almost half of these will require surgery (Butler and Lewis 1976). Enlargement of the prostate gland can disturb normal urination and can lead to infections, or even to kidney damage.

Three different surgical interventions are commonly employed in prostate surgery, depending on the severity of the problem: transurethral resection, suprapubic, and perineal procedures. The first two surgeries typically do not disturb male potency. However, the perineal procedure is the principal cause of impotence following prostatic surgery. It is important for an older man to discuss with his surgeon the type of surgery and its implications for sexual function.

Recovery from prostatic surgery usually takes up to six weeks. After surgery, semen is no longer ejaculated through the penis but is pushed back into the bladder and is later discharged in the urine. After healing occurs, the capacity to ejaculate may return in some men and fertility may also return. If surgery has been performed for cancer of the bladder or the prostate gland, the seminal vesicles that produce the fluid that mixes with the sperm may have been removed, and there will be no fluid produced at all. However, the feeling of orgasm or climax will still be present and there should be no lessening of sexual pleasure. If impotence remains and is not caused by nerve damage at the time of surgery, the probable cause is psychological, rather than physical, and we urge these men and their partners to seek counseling.

When the prostate gland is cancerous, the testes may need to be removed surgically (castration). Obviously, this is an emotionally distressing procedure. Similarly, surgery for cancer of the bladder, colon, or rectum may result in the creation of an artificial opening in the abdomen (ostomy) to allow the passage of the body's waste products into a pouch attached to the abdomen. Again, many will find this procedure embarrassing and discomforting. After such surgeries, sexual adjustment in most cases depends greatly on the understanding of one's partner and his/her willingness to make occasional adjustments. A sensitive surgeon or family doctor can also be a good source of counsel in helping the patient return to a satisfying sexual life. In many communities, self-help groups (which often meet at local community hospitals) can help tremendously in helping one deal with the problems created by radical surgical procedures, and both partners should be encouraged to attend and share their feelings and concerns. If such a group is not available in your community, write to the United Ostomy Association, Inc., 2001 W. Beverly Boulevard, Los Angeles, CA 90057, for the group nearest your community.

We have already spoken of the twin surgeries for women that have been linked to changes in sexual activity: the hysterectomy (removal of the uterus) and the mastectomy (removal of the breast). In the case of the latter procedure, attending a self-help group and talking with other women who have recovered from breast removal surgery will help the patient considerably in dealing with the emotional adjustment, as well as with such practical considerations as choosing a prosthesis, prosthetic bras, and even swimsuits. Reach to Recovery, a program sponsored by the American Cancer Society, is one such group. Many times a member of this group will be available to help counsel a woman facing mastectomy, and she will be available after surgery too. Fortunately, neither surgery needs to negate future sexual functioning following the healing period. If a major disruption in sexual activity occurs for an older woman, it will be due largely to emotional considerations that surround the surgery. After a hysterectomy, the patient should be careful to allow the vagina to heal completely before resuming intercourse; otherwise, intercourse may be painful. As we mentioned in chapter 3, after a convalescing period of several weeks, the vagina may have shrunk, but with patience, it will return to its normal size upon resumption of sexual intercourse. The period of time for healing will vary and should be discussed with the physician.

The replacement of hip and knee joints offers great hope for many arthritis sufferers. The healing process from such surgery varies, and the resumption of sexual intercourse and possible changes in position to ease the stress on the replacement joints should be discussed with the physician or surgeon. If such information has not been volunteered, the patient should ask when and how sexual activity can be resumed. Even after the recommended recovery period from joint replacement surgery, sexual partners may wish to consider some of the variations in position described in chapter 4 to prevent undue stress on the joints.

Surgery of any kind is a traumatic experience. The body takes time to heal, both from the physical trauma and from the emotional pain that may result from a significant alteration in one's body and self-image. Some older adults may find that sexual activity (where possible) aids in healing; for others it is painful or a distraction. Each individual and his or her sexual partner will need to discuss sensitively and thoughtfully how their surgery has been experienced and when they feel ready to resume regular sexual activity.

Radiation Therapy

Radiation therapy for various cancers will have varying effects on sexual function. In the case of treatment for cancers that do not affect the sexual organs directly, emotional factors related to the diagnosis of cancer itself may affect sexual feelings. Fatigue is one of the most commonly experienced side effects of radiation therapy, and this in itself may produce a marked decrease in sexual desire. When radiation therapy is directed to the pelvic area in women, patients may be advised to refrain temporarily from intercourse. Common side effects of radiation therapy to the pelvic area include decreased sexual desire and changes in the mucus lining of the vagina (which may cause shrinkage in the size of the vagina), a decrease in vaginal muscle tone, and a decrease in vaginal lubrication (National Institutes of Health 1985). These effects are similar to the normal changes caused by aging that occur in older women. After the termination of radiation therapy, sexual desire and the ability to resume sexual intercourse will return, usually within a few weeks. It may be necessary to use a water-based personal lubricant such as K-Y Jelly to increase vaginal lubrication and prevent trauma to the vaginal lining. If significant shrinking of vaginal tissues has occurred, you may need to use a dilator; you should consult your physician about these problems.

Radiation therapy to the genital area in men often produces temporary impotence that may begin two or three weeks after therapy begins and may continue for several weeks after treatment ends. Of course, such impotence may also be the result of the anxiety, worry, and decrease in sexual desire (libido) connected with the diagnosis of cancer. If a significant percentage of cells in the testes (which produce testosterone) are destroyed by radiation therapy, impotence may be permanent (Yasko 1982). If this occurs, a penile implant (prosthetic penis) is a possible alternative and should be discussed with a urologist and/or sexual counselor.

Chemotherapy

Cancer patients who are receiving chemotherapy are reported to have significant changes in sexual desire and functioning, particularly a marked decrease in libido. Even the simplest expressions of affection such as kissing may be compromised because of precautions (for example, protective isolation in the hospital) to prevent infection in patients whose immune system is suppressed by the drugs (Sarna 1981). The physical discomforts of gastrointestinal irritation, pain, and fatigue are major assaults on our sexuality. Even more damaging may be the effects of chemotherapy on one's self-image. Hair loss is frequently one of the most traumatic effects for women. Selecting an attractive wig before chemotherapy begins is extremely helpful; in some medical institutions, the American Cancer Society provides a free supply of wigs to be used by individuals undergoing treatment. An additional suggestion for both men and women who have experienced significant weight loss because of their treatment is they seek help with clothing selection and alterations to help maintain pride in their appearance.

Adjusting to Dialysis

Dialysis for the treatment of severe kidney disease is another modern therapy that may have profound effects on sexual function. At least one-third of older patients at our major medical center complain of sexual difficulties while receiving dialysis treatments. As with other forms of treatment, whether it be drugs, surgery, radiation, or chemotherapy, each individual will be affected differently. However, in the case of dialysis, men and women commonly report changes in sexual interest and in the ability to achieve orgasm. Men frequently report difficulties having an erection. As with sexual problems related to other serious illness and treatment, the causes may be physical, psychological, social, or a combination of all of these. Changes in blood chemistry often produce profound fatigue. Women frequently experience vaginal dryness, which makes intercourse uncomfortable. Men may experience changes in hormone levels that affect sexual desire and performance. Patients who are on peritoneal dialysis must deal with the appearance of a catheter in the abdomen, which may produce some of the same feelings experienced by ostomy patients and their partners. The most important effects of dialysis on sexual function may be caused by depression, which results from both physical and psychological changes caused by undergoing dialysis. These changes are similar to those we have described for other types of therapy, but because dialysis usually must be performed on a continuing basis, the adjustment in sexual habits and routines must also be long lasting. There is an excellent booklet entitled, *Sex and Dialysis*, written by Barbara Ulery. It may be ordered by sending $3.75 to Barbara Ulery, P.O. Box 462, Durango, CO 81301.

Despite the physical and emotional trauma that may be associated with surgeries and other therapies that affect our feelings about ourselves and our bodies, experience often shows that sexual activity may actually be improved after these experiences, particularly in patients who were seriously ill before surgery. It is important for both partners to understand that adjustments in sexual activity patterns require time, patience, and understanding, and above all, honest communication between partners. If a serious disruption has occurred in sexual communications, perhaps even before the onset of a serious illness, the partners may need a long time to reestablish such communication. Recognizing that sexual routines may be changed by a serious illness or its treatment will help to prevent unrealistic expectations. In some relationships, the partners may need to seek professional counseling. Even in the absence of sexual intercourse, the need for touch, intimacy, and tenderness is always most acute in times of pain or distress.

6

The Aging Mind
and Sexuality

As we noted in the first chapter, sexual response takes place "as much between the ears as between the legs." The mind plays a significant role in adult sexual functioning, and sexual health requires a foundation of good mental health.

As one reaches later adulthood or old age, a lot of "baggage" accumulated over a lifetime is brought along. Part of this baggage is our past experience with sexual feelings and activities. For some, sexual expression has been vitally important; for others, it may have been largely a necessary evil. As a rule, for those to whom sex has been important and satisfying, growing older will have a limited effect on their sexual behavior. They will do what comes naturally and brings satisfaction, unless something happens to change their situation dramatically (for example, illness or death of a spouse). For others, for whom sexuality has been unsatisfying or of lesser importance, early sexual retirement is likely to occur. Whatever the choice, it is important to keep in mind that our sexual nature goes far beyond whether or not we are sexually active at any particular point in life. More important is whether we are comfortable with the decision.

Aging in the late adult years certainly presents its own set of challenges. Health in an aging body can easily be compromised as the risk of illness increases with the advancing years. Likewise, mental health is easily threatened in the older adult. The vulnerability of the older adult to mental disease results from a combination of factors that commonly occur with aging. Physical illness, especially life-threatening illness, taxes our mental health. Losses associated with aging, such as the death of friends, relatives, or spouses, strike hard at our mental reserves. Retirement and a drop in income may produce life-style changes that are not always easy to accept emotionally. Even the physical changes of our bodies, resulting in the relative loss of strength and beauty, challenge our state of mind. Aging is a stressful process, although perhaps no more so than any other phase of human development.

Illness of any kind is distracting. The mind shifts from various problem-solving tasks associated with daily living to a preoccupation with the illness itself. An individual must manage the pain, reflect on the long-range effects of the illness, and adjust to restrictions in daily living that the illness may demand. In managing illness, the mind typically does not focus much on sexual need or desire for sexual encounter. This can be very disconcerting if one person in a partnership is ill and therefore uninterested in sexual relations while the other's normal sexual needs and interests remain alive and well. Such a relationship can easily be strained by misunderstanding.

Specific illnesses, of course, do more than distract us from sexual expression. They can, in fact, directly limit our ability to function sexually. We have covered some of these illnesses and their effects on sexual function in chapters 4 and 5. For now, we need only state that the more an illness affects our sexual capacity and the more that we value ongoing sexual activity, the more likely it is that we will experience some emotional consequences. These emotional consequences may, in turn, confound and complicate our future sexual response. For example, a man with severe prostatic disease may find that his condition reduces the pleasure associated with sexual activity, and he may experience temporary impotence. After successful treatment of the disease, it is not unusual to find the man "uncertain" and "fearful" about resuming sexual intercourse. Comparably, many women who have undergone a hysterectomy fear that they will not be able to resume normal sexual lives comfortably and successfully. The illness has caused these individuals to lose confidence in themselves as sexual beings.

The ultimate in loss of health, of course, is death. Death of a spouse or sexual partner is, naturally, highly disruptive to sexual routines. The grief typically associated with such a loss tends to reduce sexual interest and need. On the other hand, the loneliness resulting from such a loss increases our need and interest in having someone to hold us and share intimacy. Loss of a spouse is one of many losses that can trigger depression. We often feel weighed down with grief and melancholy. Breaking out of a grief reaction, particularly with renewed sexual interest, often requires the passing of the depression. Depression siphons off our *energy* and turns us inward. Successful sexual activity requires energy, sensitivity, and interest in someone beyond ourselves—our sexual partner. For example, a late middle-aged friend of ours lost his wife to cancer. For six months after her death, he grieved and experienced a heavy depression. His sexual routine was denied him. It mattered little, however, because his sexual interest virtually did not exist. Only after his depression passed did his sexual drive return and force him to deal with his sexual future.

Many factors affect our state of mind. Health, success, and feelings of personal attractiveness appear to be common variables in supporting mental health. Whether our bodies experience illness or not, they continue to change. They grow old, they grow weak. The loss of strength and beauty are factors that strongly affect self-concept. Positive self-concept is definitely part of good mental health and, correspondingly, contributes significantly to good sexual health. If we believe ourselves to be growing ugly as part of growing old, we will find it difficult to maintain an image of ourselves as sexually attractive and interesting. It is unlikely that we will remain sexually active in later life if we believe ourselves to be sexually unappealing. Unfortunately, our culture does not do a very good job of defining the relative nature of beauty with age. Not all the changes of physical aging are negative ones, and many people become more, not less, attractive. Appearance is a complex combination of many factors—body shape, posture, clothing, grooming, cosmetics, and personality—and we do have control over most of these factors as we get older. As older persons ourselves (or as related caregivers), we need to realize that beauty belongs in the eye of the beholder and that sexual interest is affected more by what is beneath the surface than what is on it.

Our mental processes are highly dependent upon our senses—sight, hearing, taste, touch, and smell. We depend on our senses for the information we use in everyday problem solving. When our senses lose some of their efficiency and acuity, we lose some of the information we need, or at least it is delayed in getting to us. Such losses often produce stress and anxiety. As a result, our judgments (decisions) may not be as good. People may misinterpret our behaviors or judgments, believing us to be senile when in fact we are experiencing sensory malfunction.

It is not uncommon to misinterpret the behavior of others when one suffers from sight and/or hearing losses. Depending upon our preexisting mental state, we can actually become paranoid, believing that others are talking about us or plotting against us. The fear and anxiety associated with such paranoia virtually eliminate the ability to see others as sexually attractive or to view intimacy as a source of solace and relief. Take the case of an older woman with failing sight and hearing loss who throughout her life harbored suspicions about people around her. Increasingly, she finds herself suspicious about her husband's faithfulness. Although unfounded, this suspicion affects her relationship with her husband. Part of this attitude includes an unwillingness on her part to continue as a sexual partner. Sensory loss, fortunately, should not physically prevent sexual encounter from occurring. Blind and deaf persons can make love as readily as can the sighted and hearing.

Our mental states do not have to be as dramatic as depression or paranoia to disrupt our sexual lives. Simple changes in our everyday lives can result in feelings of uselessness or just plain boredom. The typical signs and symptoms of real depression may be absent. In their place might be listlessness or irritability. An example is that of a man who puts away his lunch box after forty years of hard labor in a factory. Tomorrow he will not punch the time clock. A strong, virile man who once loaded hundred-pound boxes into trucks can now sleep as late as he wants to. No longer does he have a supervisor to harass him. But the welcoming feeling toward retirement is short-lived. He awakens one morning to find himself feeling old, useless, and irritable. A lifelong pattern of lovemaking on Sunday evening is ignored because he just does not feel up to it. He blames getting old for his loss of sexual interest, not realizing that the other factors contribute.

Another example is a woman who for years found her greatest pleasure in needlework. Failing eyesight because of a progressive diabetic condition makes it impossible for her to continue her hobby. Always an active and loving woman with her husband, she now finds herself out of sorts with him regularly. Her irritability is especially sharp on the occasions when they were accustomed to making love. Without really discussing the matter, the couple retires sexually, much to the disappointment of the husband and with resulting guilt in the wife.

Sexual relations between most adult sexual partners become patterned and routine. Some writers speak of this as inevitably resulting in boredom with sex. The bored sexual partners then either retire sexually, perform perfunctorily, or pursue more exciting (usually just new and different) partners. This so-called seven-year itch has been well documented. Boredom in our terms is a state of mind, a mental condition that fits somewhere between apathy and depression. The popular literature is full of prescriptions for curing this midlife crisis, espousing everything from finding new techniques to turn on one's sexual partner to renewing marital vows.

It is important to trace the origin of the state of boredom. Is it really boredom with the sexual experience or a more pervasive boredom with oneself or with one's partner? One really has not given up on sexual activity. Like eating, when treated with moderation, it is almost always a pleasant experience. So a bored person will necessarily have to take stock of the real basis for the boredom—not its symptoms. Obviously, maintaining a positive relationship with one's sexual partner is almost essential to maintaining sexual health in later life. For some older persons, admittedly, this means finding a new partner as illness and death rob them of their partners.

Another psychological phenomenon associated with older adulthood is an increased awareness of one's own mortality. When major illness strikes or a friend or a loved one our age dies, we are reminded that death will also be part of our experience—and, perhaps, sooner than we think. This mind-set, of course, can trigger in us a desire to consume as much of life as possible. In sexual terms it can drive us into promiscuous and immoderate sexual behavior. We operate as if there will be no tomorrow, often looking rather foolish in the process. Preoccupation with death, if not rationally handled, can grow into a true clinical depression. This readily occurs when one feels that there is no time to go back and experience all the pleasures one may have missed. An unhappy, sexless marriage for an aging couple may be perceived as a permanent loss, and the belief that no new beginning is really possible or worth the effort results in depression.

The most feared of all personality changes, of course, are those associated with organic brain disease. Today the most frightening of these diseases is Alzheimer's disease. While only a small percentage of older adults will ever be affected by dementias of the Alzheimer's type, those who are afflicted will demonstrate an extremely variable emotional repertoire. Irritability, crying jags, paranoia, confusion, delusions, and hallucinations may all become part of this repertoire. The disease itself may not reduce the victims' sexual appetites, but it can alter their sexual attractiveness to their partners. We would like to add a note of caution at this point. Before accepting the diagnosis of dementia or irreversible brain disease in oneself or a loved one, you should rule out all other possibilities. The scientific literature in recent years has noted that between 5 and 15 percent of older persons who were thought to be demented were actually suffering from depression (Feinberg and Goodman 1984). Once the depression was treated, the so-called dementia disappeared. The brain of the older adult is also extremely sensitive to the body's internal environment, and acute or chronic medical illness may produce behaviors that may be misinterpreted as evidence of dementia. Such physical conditions may include anemia, poorly controlled diabetes, urinary tract infections, pneumonia, congestive heart failure, kidney disease, hypothyroidism, and chronic lung disease, to name only a few. Medications, particularly sedatives or hypnotics, are another frequent cause of behavior that appears to suggest dementia. We believe that it is worth remembering the advice of the National Institute on Aging Task Force (1980): "It is crucial for health professionals, public planners, and lay persons to recognize that many curable physical and psychological diseases in the elderly produce intellectual impairment that may be hard to distinguish from irreversible brain disease" (p. 259).

For the dementias that are irreversible, little can be done, other than careful management to keep the more troublesome symptoms from getting out of hand. Many communities have support groups for families of Alzheimer's victims, and these groups provide much needed support and education. Further information may be obtained by writing to the Alzheimer's Disease and Related Disorders Association, 360 North Michigan Avenue, Chicago, IL 60601.

A brain disease can alter judgment and trigger sexual acting out (for example, open masturbation, stripping off one's clothing). Sexually based symptoms can occur even in the most prudish person, depending on the nature of the disease in the brain. The more embarrassing problems usually can be controlled through appropriate medication and good medical management, but some understanding and tolerance may be needed nonetheless. The most important thing is not to assume that such behavior somehow reflects some previously hidden vice or lack of character.

The role of our minds and emotions in maintaining sexual health in later life cannot be overstated, and it becomes even more significant in old age. The physiological urge for sex diminishes as we grow older, leaving the mind as the key "reminder" of our sexual nature. The more our minds are able to function without needless distractions, the more likely these reminders will be noticed. Where mental disease is present, one can expect disruption of sexual interest and desire. Only successful treatment of the mental disease will restore sexual health in most of these cases.

Fortunately, mental disease is the exception in old age. Mental distractions—that is, emotional disruptions—are common, however, and may temporarily disrupt our sexual health. As has been noted, many factors in old age can precipitate these emotional disruptions. All seem to have the same effect—they distract us from our sexual nature. Ironically, the best antidote to emotional stressors in our lives may be sexual activity—intimacy that provides security and comfort. Sexual health suggests that we deal with our stress and anxiety through our sexual being rather than through shelving our sexual needs and interests—if, and only if, sexual expression has served us in such reassuring fashion throughout our lives.

7

Maintaining
Personal Sexual Health

MAINTAINING sexual health takes some planning and effort at any age. In old age, when health in general becomes a bit precarious, maintaining sexual health may become even more challenging. Yet we have documented throughout this book that old age itself rarely renders older people sexual cripples. For the most part, our sexual equipment works quite adequately, even in the presence of most chronic illnesses, medical treatment, and degenerative changes of aging.

In this chapter, we would like to discuss some ideas for maintaining sexual interest and activity in later life. We are defining sexual health as the ability to maintain a level of sexual expression adequate to our needs and interests, and commensurate with the state of health of our minds and bodies. Sexual health is clearly a function of our general physical and mental health.

Maintaining Mental Health

We have argued in earlier chapters that sexual interest and responsiveness are actually more mental than physical. To focus properly on another person in a caring relationship requires freedom from serious mental distractions. For example, we have noted how difficult it is for a depressed person to seek out and invest in a love relationship. The depression turns us inward on ourselves and away from a love object. Depression empties us of our libido—our sexual energy. Depression often produces a loss of appetite, whether for food or sex.

In old age, we may find it virtually impossible to avoid depression completely, given the losses we are likely to experience. However, we can choose to succumb to losses or we can choose to deal with them. Losses can be reframed as challenges. Take the loss of physical attractiveness as it is defined in our culture: we cannot deny the wrinkles that come with age or the shifting of body fat. These are real changes. But what is their meaning? How do we choose to define such changes? We need to remember that beauty is in the eye of the beholder. Sex appeal is a mental state rather than a physical reality. Being attractive and attracting others is a quality of the whole person, not just of the face and body. As we have stated previously, sexual turn-on takes place in the mind, and sexual feelings are enhanced by sharing with a loving partner. In the depressed person, the depression erodes sex appeal far more than any physical state of the person's body.

Our task is to manage the depression, to help ourselves get beyond it. If it does not respond to self-help, then we need to seek treatment. Despite its widespread presence among the older adult community, depression responds well to treatment. Overcoming depression generally will restore sexual interests; renewed sexual interest will generate sexual responsiveness. In turn, our loving sexual experiences will help us in any future battles with depression.

Dealing with Anger

Anger is a powerful emotion that affects our sexual interest and responsiveness. When losses of loved ones and friends occur, or when we face serious illness and must take drugs or undergo treatments that assault our self-image or cause us discomfort, understandably we may become angry. Sometimes we become angry at ourselves, somehow believing that we are to blame for these misfortunes; in other cases, we may blame our illness or those who take care of us. Some people who are ill find themselves angry or resentful toward the partner who is healthy. Regardless of the reasons for it, the anger affects our ability to enjoy and share sexual feelings with another. Anger tends to feed on itself and produce even more angry feelings. Again, if you are unable to deal with and resolve these angry feelings, you may find it helpful to see a professional counselor.

Retirement from Work

Another common threat to sexual health is the mental state that may appear after retirement from work. For a career- or occupationally oriented person, retirement can be emotionally distressing. The sense of self-worth and purpose may be challenged in such people as a result of separation from long-time work colleagues and work activities. Any threat to the sense of personal worth tends to spill over into sexual life. Some people really do not feel old until they retire, and for some, when they feel old, they feel sexless. Men are particularly vulnerable to the "retirement blues." It would be interesting to know how many men sexually retire at about the same time they retire occupationally, given the possible connection between sexual vitality and a sense of personal worth and purpose.

Retirement can also change the intensity of contact between partners. The retired partner's being home and underfoot for extended periods may change the quality of a relationship—sometimes for the better, too often for the worse. Being available, of course, can create greater opportunities and occasions for lovemaking. It can also have the opposite effect by creating too much of a good thing, which may increase the opportunities for friction between the partners to build up. Most couples generally need to provide some "distance" in their relationship, so that each partner may meet some personal needs and interests without feeling consumed by the partner. Each newly retired person needs to be alerted to this danger and to make whatever adjustments are appropriate to the specific situation. This, of course, does not imply that couples who enjoy spending time together and sharing activities should not continue to do so, but pursuing hobbies and interests as individuals will often add some excitement and interest to a couple's relationship. It is never too late to take up a new hobby or to pursue intensively an interest for which there may not have been time in earlier years. For those older adults who find themselves alone, the active involvement in new interests will provide a wonderful way to meet others.

Thoughtful retirement planning that assures us ongoing purpose and place beyond our jobs will also serve as sexual health planning for later life. A host of things are yet to be done in this world that will keep us in the company of good people and help to keep that vital force alive in us—a force that we draw upon in maintaining sexual interest and responsiveness. We need to see such activities and our participation in them as valuable, not simply as "busy work" done by those who are no longer in the work force.

At any age, external events can disrupt our personal equilibrium and cause mental anguish. Many of these events are beyond our control. What we can do is learn to cope with these exigencies of life. We can develop new ways of coping and problem solving. Mental health requires mental exercise; it benefits from habits of positive thinking. Mental health also is served by sexual experiences. A loving sexual relationship is a remarkable defuser of anxiety. It is an excellent restorer of self-image and self-worth. It gives the energy needed to solve problems. In return, a restored mental equilibrium greatly facilitates sexual interest and responsiveness. At all costs, we need to avoid the "I am getting senile" mind-set. Keeping the mind exercised and staying fully invested in the world around us serves sexual health as well as mental health.

Maintaining Physical Health

Staying physically healthy is certainly a basic requirement for maintaining sexual health. Illness of any kind, at any age, is a major distraction in our lives. It demands a lot of the energy that we normally use in sexual response. A body that feels good physically responds to sexual excitement far better than does one filled with aches and pains. In the later years, good health may become even more important than the shape of our bodies as the basis for sexual attractiveness.

Staying sexually healthy implies having a life-style that promotes good physical health. This includes a sensible diet, regular exercise, restful sleep, and limited stress. We are not talking about becoming Olympic athletes. Certainly the physical demands of sexual activity are minimal. Rather, we are referring to general fitness, and, where possible, the avoidance or control of disease or illness.

Diet and Nutrition

We have discussed the importance of a balanced diet and moderate food intake. The booklet *Good Eating for the Older Adult* has helpful, easy-to-understand guidelines to sensible eating. It may be obtained by sending a check for $2.25 to the Dietary Department, University of Iowa Hospitals and Clinics, Iowa City, IA 52242. Many other nutritional guides are available from your public library, and several government publications give specific nutritional guidelines for older adults. If weight loss has been recommended, your physician, nurse, or dietitian can recommend a sensible plan to help you trim calories while maintaining good nutrition. Nutritional requirements may change as the result of an illness or treatment, and it is important to follow the dietary recommendations of your health care professional at this time. Many of our former ideas, such as very low calorie, low-carbohydrate/high-protein diets for losing weight, are no longer considered valid. For instance, we now know that adults need less protein, less fat, and more complex carbohydrates (like fruits, vegetables, and whole grain breads) to aid in weight loss and to maintain a healthy life-style. Older women need to be aware of the importance of maintaining an adequate calcium intake to help prevent osteoporosis (thinning of the bones). Specific dietary advice in this regard should be sought from health care professionals. For those who live alone, cooking nutritious meals that provide a variety of foods is often a difficult task, and such individuals often find themselves eating only what is handy and what requires the least amount of effort. Perhaps it is time for those who live alone to join forces with others and plan some "community" meals, where each contributes a portion of the meal. Such activities bring social enjoyment as well as good nutrition. Joining with one or two others in purchasing groceries often allows you to have a greater variety of fresh dairy products or produce that might otherwise spoil before one person can use them up. Those who find it difficult to follow a weight loss program alone might consider joining a group such as Weight Watchers. Any additional congregate gathering also enhances and promotes important sexual exchanges.

While we are discussing diet and nutrition, this might be a good place to mention briefly the importance of paying attention to dental health. This area is often neglected by a large number of older adults. Adding high-fiber fruits and vegetables to one's diet is a good idea, but such foods require good chewing ability. Teeth and dentures need to be in good condition to enable us to eat a variety of foods and to chew properly. In addition, an attractive smile sends a very positive message to the rest of the world. The mouth is an important source of connection between loving and sexually involved partners.

The Need for Exercise

The importance of exercise in maintaining general health as well as sexual health cannot be overemphasized. Adults who participate in a regular program of exercise often have a healthier self-image and higher self-esteem than those who do not exercise. It is important to find a form of exercise that is enjoyable, easy to do on a regular basis (at least three times per week for approximately half an hour) regardless of the weather, and does not require expensive equipment or fees. Walking briskly certainly meets all of these guidelines, and walking with a friend passes the time quickly and helps you to maintain your motivation. Many shopping malls have early morning walking groups that can be used when the weather prevents walking outdoors. Some senior centers and community recreation centers have special exercise sessions for older adults. Exercising with a group is often more fun, gives one an opportunity to meet new people, and provides a greater incentive to continue exercising (experts say that it takes about three weeks to make exercise a habit). Swimming is another excellent form of exercise, and it is especially suitable for those with severe arthritis, because the water cushions the joints. Aquatic exercising may be done even by those who cannot swim. If you do not know how to swim, it is never too late. In many cities, instructors who specialize in teaching older adults can be found.

A Good Night's Sleep

Changes in sleep patterns are often distressing as we grow older. We may find ourselves sleeping fewer continuous hours at night but taking some short naps during the day. At any age, people vary in their need for sleep. If there has been a drastic change in your sleep pattern, you might be wise to discuss this with your physician. Earlier in this chapter, we talked about depression. Excessive sleeping and feelings of fatigue despite a good night's sleep are often symptoms of depression, and they should be investigated. Although a light snack and a warm glass of milk may help you get to sleep, a large meal close to bedtime will often have the opposite effect and should be avoided. Regular exercise each day is a good aid to sleep, but vigorous exercise right before bedtime should be avoided, for it may be too stimulating. The relaxation that results from pleasurable sexual activity, either with a partner or from masturbation can be very helpful in getting to sleep. When simple measures fail or insomnia becomes threatening to one's health, it is time to seek professional help.

Stress

Although it would be desirable to be free of stressful situations that may affect our health, it is not a very realistic expectation. Since stress is a normal part of everyday life, the best course of action is to learn to deal with it and minimize its harmful effects. In earlier chapters we have talked about the benefits of sexual activity and being involved in a caring relationship, which will help protect us from anxiety and help us deal with stress. Exercise is another great stress reliever. Some exercise programs will have portions devoted to special breathing and relaxation techniques for relieving stress, or you may take a class devoted solely to relaxation techniques. *A word of caution:* if you are taking any medications to lower blood pressure, please check with your physician and tell your exercise instructor before engaging in such sessions. Many relaxation technqiues are designed to help you lower your pulse rate and blood pressure, and this may be dangerous if you are also taking a medication that does the same thing.

Illness and Sex

When illness does occur, sexual health is best protected by quickly curing or containing the illness, if possible. For instance, a diabetic whose blood sugar gets out of control may face sexual complications, especially men, who may suddenly experience impotence. The same diabetic whose blood sugar is kept normal can expect his sexual response to be normal. As we noted in chapter 5, the treatment of a disease or our feelings about the disease and treatment may pose as much of a threat to our sexual well-being as the disease itself. Once again, we need to work closely with our physicians and pharmacists to monitor any sexual side effects from drugs and report problems promptly. Although some health care professionals still suffer from ageism when it comes to viewing older adults as sexually interested and active, in fairness to those who care for our health, we must realize that they are more likely to be experts in treating our disease rather than in dealing with our sexual concerns. If we believe that our sexual concerns are not being dealt with effectively, we need to discuss this with those who care for us and ask for further help.

Where chronic diseases are already present (for example, hypertension, diabetes, arthritis, and so forth), close medical management of these conditions is essential to good sexual health. We must assume some of this responsibility by using available health resources properly. Maintaining a healthy life-style will help greatly in minimizing some of the effects of chronic disease.

Appearance and Sex Appeal

At any age, good hygiene and grooming add to our sex appeal. To believe that looks no longer count as one gets older is to fail to understand the psychology of aging. Vanity does not disappear with age and, in some cases, becomes more dominant in later life. Older adults often seem to make more small talk about their bodies than they do about the weather.

Just as we notice "health" in a person, we tend to take note of personal appearance. We are attracted to people who seem to care about themselves. We like to see people comfortably well dressed. Fortunately, being well dressed is *not* the same as being expensively dressed. An expensive wardrobe does not necessarily buy us sex appeal. Grooming, hygiene, and wardrobe are all part of what Gordon Alport (1955) calls our "ego-extension." They are signs of what is inside us. A sexually alive person will be likely to give off *signs* of sexual interest through hygiene, grooming, and clothing.

In old age, grooming and hygiene and even what we wear are not always under our control. A frail or infirm person in a nursing home or one who is dependent upon a caregiver at home must depend on others to attain these personal care goals. The performance of this role in long-term care facilities may be the institution's major contribution to the sexual health of its residents. For example, we know a very frail woman in a nursing home who was little more than skin and bones. She had lost a leg because of poor circulation, and her hands and arms were severely deformed by rheumatoid arthritis. Yet she was always well dressed and beautifully groomed. Her gray hair, carefully coiffured, had remained silky and nicely textured. Even with all the bodily damage, it was not her frailty that caught your eye when you met her, but her exceptional appearance. Instead of repelling others because of the extent of the damage to her body, she projected quite a positive image. Obviously, this meant that nursing home staff members appreciated the importance of her appearance to her and to those around her. We would like to suggest to our readers that they may be at some point in the position of having to choose a care facility for themselves or for a relative. We think that it is important to look at the grooming of the residents in such facilities as one measure of how the staff members view the significance of a positive self-image for their residents.

For those who are still able to attend to their own grooming and clothing needs but are on a slim budget, there are many ways to maintain their appearance. Many older adults have grown children and grandchildren who are often at a loss for gift ideas on birthdays and holidays. It might be helpful for such elders to suggest that family members pool their resources for a gift certificate at a favorite department store, or an intergenerational shopping trip may even be enjoyable. Do not overlook the nicer consignment shops that may be found in many medium to large cities. High quality clothes for both men and women may often be found for very low prices. If you take the time to become friendly with the store personnel, they frequently will keep you in mind when items come in and will let you have "first pick." For professional hair care for both men and women, a nearby beauty school will usually charge a very affordable price for its services, and it may even have an additional discount for senior citizens. Many cosmetic stores will have free demonstrations and will apply the newest colors and products in makeup. Even if you do not choose to buy what you have tried, such a session will help you decide on the most flattering colors and techniques that can be duplicated with less expensive products. Discount stores and catalogues may offer clothing and makeup at substantial savings. The American Association of Retired Persons has a catalogue of pharmaceutical products that also includes makeup and personal care items for both men and women at discount prices. This catalogue is sent to members. When we talk about hygiene, grooming, and attractive clothing for older adults, we are talking to men as well as women. Many older men may feel that it is somehow less than masculine to be concerned with such things as hairstyle, skin care, and other details of grooming, but personal care and pride in one's appearance is important for both sexes.

Appearance goes beyond our looks and clothes. It extends into our immediate social environment. Our sexual responsiveness is an aroused phenomenon. Sometimes, particularly when we are young, it is purely hormone-driven and comes from the inside. More often it is teased into response by the conditions and situations we experience. Many of these situations can be brought within our control. For instance, we can arrange a candlelight supper once in a while; we can add fragrant flowers to match the fragrance of our perfume; we can add the right music to touch off our feelings. These romantic gestures are as appropriate and important for older adults as they are for younger ones. The mechanical aspects of lovemaking are perhaps given too much emphasis in our culture. However, some variations in lovemaking, including occasionally changing times and places, can keep sexual relations fresh and alive, even for long-time partners.

Creative Sexual Response

Staying sexually healthy also means knowing when and how to make adjustments and adaptations in our sexual response to cope with age-related changes in our bodies. The first step is simply knowing how sexual response can be compromised by the aging of our bodies. This knowledge should reduce the likelihood of premature sexual retirement because of ignorance. The second step is learning to solve problems. When age or illness present a roadblock to our sexual response, we need to find a detour. An incredible number of such exigencies can occur in late life sexuality, and it is beyond the scope of this book to address all of them. However, we will present a few examples to assure our readers that there are many alternate routes toward gaining a satisfying sexual life available to a person whose sexual response may be compromised somewhat by age-related changes.

As we discussed earlier, a common problem in older men is the time factor in experiencing an erect (hard) penis. As we have explained, the process of congesting blood in the penis takes a little bit to a lot longer, depending on the individual's age and state of health. Obviously it is necessary to allow sufficient time for lovemaking to avoid an occasion of impotency. Such patience will be most tolerated when both partners understand and appreciate the reason for allowing adequate time for lovemaking. A little more imagination in arousing sexual excitement also helps. For some men, hand massaging of the penis is very important; for others, kissing or nipple massage may be even more important. Some couples have discovered that using a vibrator to stimulate the sensitive areas of the body *gently* (particularly the underside of the penis or the clitoris) will bring about sexual arousal. If this method is used, it should not be used too frequently or for too long, for it is possible to irritate the genitals, particularly if the skin is dry or tender. The genitals can be lubricated with K-Y Jelly or a soft handkerchief can be placed between the vibrator and the area being stimulated. With any of these suggested activities, which may not have been a part of previous sexual activity, open and honest communication between sexual partners is important. Unfortunately, among older couples, such communication typically may not have been part of their lovemaking experience for many years (if ever), so it is time for a change.

Knowing that the penis may not achieve the hardness required for penetration, a thoughtful partner can help by assisting a somewhat soft penis into the vagina (this is sometimes referred to as "stuffing"). Entry, even partial entry, will often serve to harden the penis sufficiently to complete intercourse. The female partner may have to work a little harder than usual if her male partner is having such difficulties. Both partners should also remember that it is the end of the penis and the clitoris and opening to the vagina that are most sensitive, and deep penetration of the penis into the vagina is not necessary in order for the female partner to experience pleasure and satisfaction.

There is really no failure in sexual encounters if one accepts the idea that a sexual connection is more than just a completed act of intercourse. Touching, kissing, holding, or simply being close together and talking about feelings are all sexual experiences that may be thought of as ends in themselves. They afford both partners a good feeling and loving connection.

For some couples, oral-genital contact can serve as an alternative to strictly genital contact, depending on their respective views about this type of sexual contact. A woman for whom sexual intercourse is painful may welcome oral contact. For a male, oral-genital contact may help him to achieve an erect penis. In old age we may need to add to our repertoire of lovemaking techniques, assuming that we are comfortable with any additions. Again, communciation between partners is very important.

For those who suffer from arthritis or low back pain, where pain is being experienced in conventional or traditional patterns of sexual intercourse, some experiments with altered positions or approaches to intercourse may help (see chapter 4). Other suggestions for those with arthritis include the use of a pain relief medication timed to be most effective during sexual intercourse, exercises to relax the joints, a warm bath or shower before sexual activity (perhaps with a partner), and massaging of the painful areas. Obviously, these approaches may also be enjoyed by those who do not have arthritis.

As a rule, if people are comfortable with their sexuality and are honest with themselves, they can find a way around most pains or physical limitations to make a satisfying sexual connection. Lovemaking in these cases simply takes the same ingenuity that we apply to other tasks, such as getting in and out of the bathtub, or figuring out how to put on our shoes and socks as we grow frail. It may look funny to an outsider, but as long as it works, that is the important thing.

Professional Counseling

Throughout this book, we have advised professional counseling when either emotional or physical barriers to sexual expression cannot be overcome by the partners themselves. Sex therapy may be offered by professionals in many different fields, including psychiatry, psychology, social work, medicine, and nursing, as well as by members of the clergy. At the present time, the field of sex therapy is not regulated, and it is possible for anyone to call him- or herself a sex therapist. Even among highly qualified sex therapists, very few specialize in sexual problems of older adults. Masters, Johnson, and Kolodny (1986) suggest some general guidelines for selecting a sex therapist, including seeking one through sex therapy centers affiliated with universities, medical schools, or hospitals, and seeking referrals from a local physician and medical society. To their suggestions we might add that you ask specifically for counselors who specialize in working with the elderly. Several medical centers around the country now have special geriatric and gerontology education centers for training health care personnel to address the sexual concerns of older adults as part of their approach to health care.

Masturbation

A common issue in late life sexuality is the temporary or permanent loss of a partner. An alternative means of sexual expression, with or without a partner, is masturbation. Self-arousal can provide sexual pleasure and may lead to orgasm. Masturbation thus can relieve sexual tension that may have built up in the absence of sexual intercourse. It may also help to maintain physical sexual responsiveness (to maintain the shape of the vagina for women, or to maintain the production of semen in men) when regular sexual intercourse is not possible. Masturbation is a common sexual practice among persons of all ages and may serve as an alternative means of sexual expression for partners who are not interested in or who are unable to have sexual intercourse. Like all modes of sexual expression, our attitudes toward this type of activity will influence its ability to satisfy us, but there are no physical or psychological arguments against masturbation. Surveys of older adults indicate that masturbation is a very common sexual practice, particularly among older women. In their book *The Widow's Guide to Life* (Fisher and Lane 1981) the authors comment that "the alternatives to masturbation are walking around grumpy, taking tranquilizers, or jumping into bed with the first available man" (p. 108).

In truth, maintaining sexual health in old age is perhaps more tied to our zest for life than any other single factor. If we want to live fully in our later years, then in all likelihood we will maintain active sexual interests. All of our appetites for living stay strong and give direction to the ways in which we invest our energies. We seek out friends, pursue social activities, and delight in the activities of daily living, among which we shall include meeting our sexual needs. As older persons, we have the advantage of not being driven by our sexual needs as younger people sometimes are. We can become more patient lovers, discovering the aspects of sexuality that go beyond sexual intercourse.

We suspect that some older adults may come to appreciate their sexuality for the first time in the later years. Relieved of the fears of pregnancy or the stress of performance, couples can relax as sexual partners and simply share a loving relationship with one another.

This brings us to the final point that we must make before leaving this chapter. Maintaining sexual health requires us to maintain at least one loving relationship. This is not always easy. Even with a long-time spouse or lover, we rarely manage a lifetime without some conflicts. Some of these conflicts may be the result of some truly unfortunate things we did at an earlier period in our relationships. Serious conflicts often produce emotional scars and lingering resentments. These present serious obstacles to healthy sexual expression in later life. Sexual health may ultimately require us to make one of the most adult responses required of human beings: forgiveness and understanding. Rarely will the unforgiving be happy in their old age. The satisfaction of being able to inflict unhappiness on another human being will never compare to the satisfaction of making another person happy. Forgiveness may ultimately be the price we pay for sexual health in later life.

8

Sex, the Older Adult, and Institutional Environments

A married patient in a long term care facility shall be assured privacy for visits by his or her spouse, and married inpatients may share a room unless medically contraindicated and so documented by the attending physician in the medical record. . . . [I]f a patient is found to be medically incapable of understanding, these rights and responsibilities devolve to the patient's sponsor. . . . The patient may associate and communicate privately with persons of his choice . . . unless medically contraindicated (as documented by his physician in the medical records) (Wharton 1981, 100–101).

O LDER adults may find themselves in many types of institutional settings, ranging from hospitals to prisons. However, in discussing sexual health in later adulthood, two basic living environments concern us: the senior citizen housing facility and the nursing home. The likelihood of an aging person's spending time in one or both of these environments is increasing greatly.

Currently 5 percent of the elderly reside in congregate housing facilities, which range from small apartment complexes to large, multiapartment high rises. Most are located in urban areas, although smaller, progressive communities now often manage a facility or two. Most of these facilities have received some financial support through a federal or state government financing program, with a mix of local, government-administered operations and both private for-profit and not-for-profit sponsors.

Nearly a quarter of all older persons will spend at least some part of their later adulthood in a long-term care facility (a nursing home). Roughly 5 percent of those over sixty-five, 1.35 million persons, will call such a facility home in their final year. The nursing home industry covers a wide range of categories from residential care facilities to skilled nursing facilities. The majority of elderly persons reside in intermediate care facilities (ICFs), where only moderate levels of nursing care are provided.

Very few institutional environments are designed with the concept in mind that older people are or will be active sexually. As a physical plant, the congregate housing facility offers largely basic shelter—a place. Spaces for congregate (shared) living are limited, since the government funding agencies usually do not provide loan money for such amenities. Except in selected rural areas, the congregate housing facility is often built on the least desirable (inexpensive) tracts of land. The outcome physically is a less than appealing environment, certainly not what we would call a sexually inviting environment.

Even more sexless is the environment in the nursing home, which looks more like a hospital ward than a home. The available space is usually partitioned off as sleeping rooms. Common spaces are few, and these areas are generally both cluttered and crowded. Even where efforts at interior decorating are made, the outcome looks like a stereotype of an "old folks' home," rather than like a lively, sexy environment. Nursing homes should fight hard to keep from looking like the last stop for the dying, rather than places for the very old to live.

Buildings themselves, however, are not the cause of the problem. More at issue is the administrative milieu that is created and the type of programming that is offered in the facility. When one or both of these fail to acknowledge the sexual nature of their residents, the living environment drops to the basic provision of bed and board, and some "care."

The power of these facilities over the lives and self-concepts of the elderly residents cannot be overstated. Few residents dare complain about problems for fear of losing what minimal amenities they have. Nevertheless, sexual health should not be regarded as a luxury but as a necessity. Like food and medicine, touch, intimacy, and love are essential to the diets of the older adult. Sensory stimulation, associated with loving care, may well be the highest-priority need of older persons living in institutional environments. Many of the older adults in nursing homes have few or no family members or friends and are completely dependent upon the staff members for gestures of touch and caring and validation of their sexual identity. Nursing home personnel need to understand, respect, and appreciate the sexual nature of the residents and to be nonjudgmental. In our state, the average age of nursing home staff members is only twenty-two; many of these young adults are not completely comfortable with their own sexuality, and they view the sexuality of the elderly with a less than sympathetic eye particularly those who are chronically ill or disabled.

In congregate facilities, older adults are likely to live alone and to be lonely apartment dwellers lost in a crowd of look-alikes. In the nursing home, loneliness is felt even under conditions where privacy has become a past luxury. Having a roommate hear you flush the toilet is a far cry from the intimacy of someone tenderly holding you.

Promoting sexual health in an institutional environment begins with the obvious: the awareness of the ongoing sexual nature of the residents. Administrators and program staff should act from the assumption that at least some of the residents are sexually active or would like to be, and secondly, that sexual activity for them is, with few exceptions, therapeutic and health giving. For others who wish to remain sexually retired or for whom illness is severe, the need to be acknowledged as sexual beings, to have their gender recognized and appreciated remains, as does the even more dramatic need for ongoing psychosensory stimulation.

Where does one begin? Perhaps the most tangible action that can be pursued is to change the physical environment itself. Added privacy is always important if sexual activity is to be made possible. Creatively finding or designing such spaces, even where congregate space is limited, is always possible.

A thoughtful interior design plan that adds a sensuous quality to the environment is helpful. Pictures on the wall say a lot about how the aged are viewed in a particular environment. What about some pictures that depict older people in touch and in love with one another, even pictures that allow for reminiscence about the "active" past? Soft carpeting, quiet spaces, and mellow lighting would provide a welcome retreat from the harsh, hospital-like, institutional appearance that both congregate facilities and nursing homes typically present.

The outside areas are just as important. Quiet retreats, gardens, nooks, water fountains, and pools are all sensual expressions. Nursing homes have the advantage here in that many have considerable amounts of green space. Some attractive landscaping is possible. Congregate housing facilities are frequently set on asphalt parking lots along urban freeways, affording little hope for an attractive outside area. Even if space permits, many elderly persons are afraid to leave their apartments in some urban areas.

Through no fault of the institutional environments themselves, the demographics of the older adults do little to facilitate sexual health. In congregate living facilities, women outnumber men by nearly three to one, and in nursing homes by as many as four or five to one. In effect, nature has at least for the time being feminized old age. The sexes have always found the time and place to gather by gender, even when cultural arrangements did not particularly encourage such segregation. However, the ambience that is found where the sexes are mixed environments (as opposed to same sex environments) seems to be more positive and healthy for most people than it is in environments where people are segregated by sex. One only needs to observe what happens in a nursing home when a handful of young men from a local college visit, or, likewise, when a group of older male volunteers from the local VFW drops by. Sexual, or at least sensual, energy is released, and the whole atmosphere comes alive. Teasing, joking, and flirting become welcomed natural encounters. If the event is preplanned, the residents will take great pains in looking their best.

One must remember that most of the staff members serving the aging female residents are themselves female. Many if not most of the volunteers active in congregate/nursing home facilities are also female. The message is clear: administrators should concentrate on hiring more male staff, volunteer coordinators should try to recruit more male volunteers, and activity coordinators should use more male volunteers in their programming. Ironically, the VA hospitals and veterans' homes are filled largely with men, whereas surrounding non-public nursing homes are filled with women.

A major force in promoting sexual health in institutional environments rests with the personnel who plan the recreational activities. Two different approaches can be followed in such program design. As with the interior design of the facility, one can program to meet the interests of "old folks" in an "old folks' home." This becomes something of a self-fulfilling prophecy: you give the old folks what you think they want, and they want what they think you have to give. There is no measure of *growth* or movement in such a plan. An alternative approach is to program for the residents much as you would for yourself—by giving them lively adult programming. In keeping with this view, programming that recognizes and facilitates the sexual nature of the participants can be emphasized. An exercise class, for example, can stretch and tone the muscles, maintaining function in aging limbs. Yet it can do more. By mixing the sexes in the group arrangements and by planning some program-related physical touch or contact, something more than pure exercise can result.

Meals in congregate facilities, when prepared by the institution, tend to take on an institutional quality. Even the routine of seating rarely varies, and somehow the men end up sitting together, as do the women. The table settings are often drab and hardly stimulating to the appetite. The consequence is uneventful if not boring meals. Eating is and has been historically a prelude to lovemaking. Mealtime could be used as the most important program time in the institution's day. But it needs some pizzazz—some atmosphere. Every once in a while, we need to dress up and eat by candlelight. The point is, we need a sexy meal even if there is no sex. The atmosphere may help us relive some important sensual moments in our past. To relive is to experience, to stay alive. Especially in a nursing home, this is terribly important. Such small amenities as flowers (not necessarily fresh if the cost is prohibitive) and candles on the table do not cost any more than the deplorable and demeaning kindergarten-type decorations that we have encountered in many nursing homes. Creating attractive, adult decorations can be incorporated into a crafts program as well.

Speaking of atmosphere, one of the nicer developments in congregate facilities is the experiment with the cocktail hour. A glass of beer or wine (or even a nonalcoholic equivalent), the drawing together, and the touching of glasses can contribute to sexual health. A small amount of alcohol can serve as an aphrodisiac for most moderate drinkers, which is usually the case with older persons living in congregate facilities. Given the antiaphrodisiac effects of most medications that many older people take, it only seems fair that such people be permitted an occasional drink if no medical reason to prohibit it exists. Unfortunately, many institutions still fail to allow such a basic amenity to their very adult residents. If alcohol must be prohibited for medical or philosophical reasons, even the serving of fruit juices in wine glasses adds a certain ambience to an ordinary occasion.

A rather interesting film called *Rose By Any Other Name* portrays an older couple who seek each other out in a retirement home. When they choose to share a bed, the home's administrator blows the whistle. The film shows the sadness created when the two elderly people, without each other's nocturnal company, reexperience loneliness. In any institutional environment, there are always "events" that take place. Sometimes they are in violation of the rules, sometimes they are precipitants of new rules, and just as often, they are overlooked. Some of these events are sexual in nature: a male resident may touch a female resident on the breast, a female resident may masturbate in a public area, a resident may make a sexual suggestion to a staff person, and so forth. What is the proper response? Categorically, an *improper* response is one in which the sexual act is denied or belittled. In such cases, it does not matter whether the older person is fully aware of his or her behavior, or whether the behavior is compromised by illness and age. Some sexual activity, of course, is inappropriate and the resident needs to be assisted in finding more privacy or in finding a more acceptable way to fulfill these needs. However, the fact that the event took place indicates the need for sexual expression in the older person. Even in congregate living settings, where residents are generally more vigorous, there can be sex scandals—which to most of us are hardly scandalous. Sensitive, thoughtful, and nonrigid responses to these events are extremely valuable in maintaining an ambience of sexual health in the institution.

With more and more older people spending an extended period of their lives in an institutional environment, we need to encourage the staff members and administrators in these institutions to recognize the lifelong sexual nature of the older adult—no matter how advanced in age.

9

How Families
Influence Sexuality
in Later Life

S EXUALITY is a private matter. Unfortunately, this is perhaps less true
than we would like it to be. In the case of the very young and
the very old, sexuality often becomes a family matter.

In this chapter, we will explore three different types of family interest in the sexuality of an older person: the highly appropriate interest of a spouse or regular sexual partner; the sometimes questionable
interest of adult children and relatives; and the correspondingly questionable interest of friends, peers, and neighbors. Our purpose is to
suggest ways to avoid or handle undesirable but common intrusions
by others into one's sexual life.

For older adults, perhaps nothing is more demeaning than to have
others question the appropriateness of active sexual interest and activity in their lives. Having been sexual throughout our entire adult lives
and having been accepted as such, the arrival of a few wrinkles and
gray hairs should not be the basis for others to assume that we are
ready for voluntary sexual retirement. Nor should the continued intimacy of two elderly persons be an occasion for joking or laughter.
We never outgrow the need to be loved or touched, unless this need
never developed in our adult lifetime or was damaged somehow in the
course of our development.

The Influence of the Partner

Sexuality typically involves a partnership; for most of us, that partner is a spouse. Just as our sexual rhythms were different at various stages throughout our lives, our sexual interest and abilities may be compromised in old age. If sexual expression has been an important part of our lives in earlier years, it is likely to continue to be important as we grow older. However, a painful illness, severe body disfigurement, an unhappy marital relationship, or a limited interest in sex throughout life may serve as an occasion for choosing to sexually retire. This may produce a situation of involuntary sexual retirement for the partner. In some cases, of course, a couple will make a mutual decision to sexually retire and will be fully agreed upon the chosen course of action. They can continue to love and care for one another without any loss of closeness.

However, if one partner suddenly decides to retire sexually, it can put a significant strain on the spousal relationship. This is particularly true if the retirement is used as an expression of anger or dislike toward the partner. Where the unilateral decision is not used as a weapon in the relationship, it may have various consequences. If the spouse has indicated his or her decision and listened to arguments by the partner, the relationship can survive, even if the choice is not mutually popular. In some instances, the partner may not prefer the choice, but may not mind it all that much. Ideally, except for genital sexual intercourse, other forms of intimacy may well continue, which will help maintain the bond between the couple.

If the decision is unpopular, the nonretiring partner may reestablish some sort of sexual life or outlet such as masturbation or a relationship with another partner. If this is discreet and/or acceptable to the retired partner, it could be a defensible solution to the problem created by the sexual retirement of one sexual partner, particularly when the other spouse or partner is mentally or physically incapacitated.

As with the reasons for any other form of retirement, the reasons behind the decision to retire sexually should be explored and understood. In many situations the decision is an unnecessary and unfortunate one. For example, some women have been known to retire sexually following the removal of a breast (mastectomy) because they felt embarrassed by the disfigurement. Or an older man may suddenly retire sexually because of an instance of impotency; he may hope to avoid the risk of repeating such an occurrence. These are situations where counseling should be pursued before a decision becomes final. Again, open communication and discussion with one's sexual partner is essential in making these decisions.

When a spouse dies or a couple separates or divorces and loss of a lifelong sexual partner occurs, sexual retirement may be involuntary at first and later become voluntary. In later life, the availability of other partners, especially for women, is a real problem. The research findings regarding the somewhat high rate of masturbation among older adults suggest that sexual needs and interests continue, even when a partner is not available. A widow or widower may feel guilty or embarrassed about pursuing a new sexual partner at this stage of life, especially if those around her or him are not supportive. This may lead to the decision to retire sexually. However, sexual health is generally best achieved when and where the interested widow or widower is able to reestablish a meaningful sexual relationship with a new partner. Surveys of sexual interest among older persons show that many elders would welcome such an opportunity.

Starting to court again is indeed awkward for a long-married person who has been in a monogamous relationship, as younger divorced people will attest. All of the issues of courtship that face younger persons must also be faced by older ones. Some older adults may question of the appropriateness and morality of sexual activity outside of marriage. Such questioning may occur not only after the death of a spouse, but also in situations where marriage is not possible, as in the case of one partner in the marriage becoming totally incapacitated or perhaps institutionalized. It is not easy to change the habits and convictions of a lifetime, but current social attitudes may allow us to rethink our views and permit us to seek a satisfying sexual relationship, even if marriage to the current sexual partner is not a consideration.

In old age an even greater loss of confidence may occur in feeling sexually attractive and interesting to a potential partner. As one will soon rediscover, courtship at any age is as exciting and challenging as it is frustrating and discomforting at times. It is a far better state of affairs than simply marking time until life's end. As we discussed in chapter 3, older men and women may find that abstinence from sexual intercourse for a relatively long period of time may cause difficulties in restarting a sexual relationship because of physical changes associated with aging. Again, we emphasize the need for both partners to understand and communicate if such problems arise.

Family Influences

Many stories are told about the reactions of children and close relatives to the ongoing sexuality of an elderly parent (or relative), especially if the parent is a widow or widower. Many children have their own feelings about the nature of loyalty to a deceased spouse. Some children treat a parent who has reestablished a sexual relationship as if he or she were having an open extramarital relationship. They will do everything to make the parent feel guilty and give up the relationship. The motives for this negative intrusion may vary. Frankly, some children may fear that remarriage will ultimately affect their inheritance or that the new partner will steal away the affections of their surviving parent. Many adult children may be shocked at the whole idea of sexual activity on the part of an older parent who they imagine has outgrown sexual needs. They may view their parent's sexuality as bordering on deviant behavior.

If the parent has a chronic illness or is in a nursing home, the children may fear that the parent's health will be jeopardized by late life sexual activity. Adult children typically are even less knowledgeable about later life sexuality than are elders themselves.

Other relatives, particularly siblings, who are usually older themselves, may be jealous of a brother's or sister's opportunity or ability to maintain an active sexual life. This jealously may be expressed openly as resentment or more covertly through attempts to make their relative feel guilty about being sexually active. Often a relative who is also a widow or widower will step forward to commisserate with and comfort someone who has lost a partner. Such a relative will often fill in for the absence of the partner and eventually may grow to need this relationship to stabilize his or her own life situation. When the object of this attention finds a new "outside" companion, the relative experiences the hurt of rejection. The person who is at the center of the situation is in the double bind of building a sexual relationship with a new partner at the expense of losing the support of a highly valued sibling or other relative.

There are no simple solutions to these problems. One must make a choice based on one's own needs to be an independent person and then work to reduce the costs of this choice. In the case of adult children who are greatly concerned about their future inheritance should the surviving parent remarry, premarital contracts may satisfy all the parties concerned. Such arrangements help to forestall any accusations that the intended spouse is simply a fortune hunter. Elders can reassure their adult children, siblings, and other relatives that the bonds of affection will not be severed by the new relationship, and that the new relationship does not represent a loss of love and respect for the former spouse. However, it is also important for adult children and relatives to recognize that the man or woman who chooses to remarry or begin a new relationship is entitled to be recognized as a whole person, not simply as the remaining half of a couple. Perhaps the blending of family members that has developed because of the frequency of divorce in the younger generation will serve as a model for adult children and their older parents.

It is important to keep in mind that not all marriages have been happy ones. Widows and widowers can have mixed emotions about the loss of their spouses. This may be particularly true if the surviving spouse filled the burdensome role of longtime caregiver to the deceased, or if one or both spouses had chosen to endure an unhappy marriage for religious or other reasons. The opportunity to explore and build new relationships may be a real source of future motivation for the surviving parent to build a new life. Children, friends, and relatives should encourage the older person to build such relationships. Doing so could be a major step toward developing and maintaining mental as well as sexual health.

Some adult children and even some widowed older adults may feel that being sexually attracted to another person or considering remarriage symbolizes disloyalty to the deceased spouse. A friend of ours who is a minister told us that when he performs a marriage ceremony for a couple whose spouses have died, he views the willingness of the couple to enter into the new relationship as a tribute to their former spouses. It symbolizes the good feelings that they had about their former marriages.

On the other hand, widows or widowers who choose to maintain their loyalties to a deceased spouse should not necessarily be criticized for doing so. While such attachments to a deceased person can be neurotic, most are natural efforts to hold on to something that has been important in the life of the surviving spouse. The memories may serve to keep a person going. Part of the memories may well include remembering some of the good sex. Such reminiscing is actually a form of our sexual experience and may contribute to sexual health in later life.

Not all adult children and relatives are threatened by a widowed parent or relative who has established a new sexual partnership. Those families who truly support their elderly relative's best interests may welcome and rejoice in the reality that the elder has been able to reestablish a sexual life. They will see this as a healthy development. In some cases, they will be especially happy that another person will be available to help their parent or relative deal with the future dependencies that may be a part of old age. They will welcome the new partner as an addition to the potential support system of their older parent or relative.

A substantial number of elderly persons live in the home of a child or near relative. For those older adults who are sexually active or who maintain a close relationship with someone "outside" the family, the pursuit of privacy in the home can be a real challenge. We mention this to alert supportive family members of the need to provide their relative with a level of privacy that could accommodate an ability to remain sexually active. Obviously, the size and structure of the family home will be a factor, given that other members of the family will also be competing for privacy. If the finances of either the family or the elderly relative permit, the possibility of building or remodeling private quarters might be considered.

The same issue of providing privacy for the older adult is present in the "shared-home" living arrangements that have become popular. The older adult may share a home with persons of various ages, as a mutual social or economic benefit. These benefits, however, must not come at the expense of privacy or constraints on the sexual life of the older person, and a frank discussion about respecting privacy among those who share such residences should take place. This is not too different from the current agreements among young adult roommates who want privacy with their special friends or lovers and agree to certain arrangements to accommodate the need for privacy.

When family interference becomes obstructive to the older person's sexual life, outside counseling may be needed; if such a resource is not available, a good heart-to-heart talk about one's right of self-determination is in order. Older adults may need to draw the line about what is right and appropriate for themselves and clearly and unequivocally communicate this to family members. To give in passively to negative intrusions of this sort can lead to unfortunate resentments and to the deterioration of very important family relationships. Those who are in a position to counsel also need to be clear about the importance of sexuality in later life and the right of sexual self-determination for older persons.

Friends and Neighbors

Whether we like it or not, nonfamily members (friends and neighbors) may have a great interest in our sexual lives. Since most people in the older age cohorts are reluctant to discuss their sexual lives as a friendship or neighborhood matter, they can expect those around them to do some conjecturing about their private lives. We have to expect and live with a certain amount of this curiosity. Rather than necessarily being damaging, such gossip could be complimentary.

The situation is most likely to be one in which friends or neighbors have shared with and comforted a widowed person and partially filled in for the loss of a partner. If the neighbor or friend is not involved with a sexual partner or is sexually retired, he or she has the comfort of sharing the "burden" with the bereaved person. This works, of course, until one or the other chooses to "come out of retirement" and starts spending time with a sexual partner. The resentment that may be experienced by the person who feels left out is often expressed in the form of criticism of the presumed sexual activities of the friend. Widows or other unattached persons who have been part of a social group made up of those also without current partners often report that they suddenly find themselves excluded from former activities once they enter into a sexual relationship. Neighbors may also take the position that a widow should remain faithful to the deceased spouse and may view a new relationship as disloyal or immoral. In an older, stable neighborhood, an unwritten cultural code to this effect may even exist. Neighbors can be cruel, closing doors and friendships to another who violates local standards. Serious courtship can be greatly complicated by overly attentive neighbors.

We have briefly described the situation where one partner in the relationship is totally incapacitated and is in an institution. This raises more than just the issue of how the remaining partner is to satisfy his or her own sexual needs. Many elderly persons in this situation tell us that even though their spouse or partner is totally incapable of any kind of response or relationship, family members and friends view the "well" partner as still married and expect that individual to conform to society's expectations for married persons. Such individuals often find themselves in a situation where they are excluded socially from the ranks of both the married and unmarried.

Of course, new friendships with persons of the opposite sex may develop in later life (especially for older widowed adults), which form with the understanding that they will remain nonsexual. Both friends may express a need for companionship, but out of respect for a deceased spouse or to simplify the new relationship, the two individuals may agree to keep their relationship platonic. This can be a highly appropriate decision if it truly reflects the wishes of the pair. Sex is not essential to human bonding or caring, as many celibates and saints have proved. And as we have emphasized repeatedly, sex is far more than sexual intercourse. In fact, all human relationships are sexual, simply because sex is an integral part of a person's humanness, and it cannot be separated out in a relationship.

In this brief chapter, we have tried to describe to our readers the public nature of the private expression of personal sexuality. We need to be aware of its existence and to be prepared to handle it when it becomes intrusive. We also need to treat others as we wish to be treated. Perhaps it is best to be honest and open with those around us. How we choose to handle our sexual needs in old age is our business, period, and it remains a private and personal matter, unless we choose to make it otherwise. Likewise, we should respect others of our peers who have voluntarily chosen to retire sexually and sympathize with those for whom it has been involuntary. Sexual health does not necessarily require active genital sexual activity. It does require acceptance of our sexual nature, awareness of our needs, and making the right choice for ourselves (and our partners, where they exist).

10

Same Sex Relationships

THROUGHOUT this book we have discussed sexual feelings and activities as something that typically takes place between partners.
We have carefully chosen the word *partner* rather than *spouse*, since
sexual relationships may be established with someone other than a spouse
and/or with someone of the same sex. We have also referred to sexuality as something more than genital contact or intercourse. Sexuality may be expressed through feelings toward another person, through
gentle touch, or even through a means as indirect as correspondence.
It is our brain more than our hormones that tells us when some manner of human connection is sexual.

In this chapter, we would like to discuss the issue of sexual relationships between older adults of the same sex. In his book, *Gay and Gray*,
Raymond Berger (1982) has written that as gay people—homosexuals
and lesbians—grow old, they retain their preference for persons of the
same sex. They also must adapt their sexuality to the aging process
in ways very similar to those of heterosexual couples. Gay as well as
straight elderly people must face their fears about the loss of sexual
attractiveness, the death or illness of a sexual partner, or diminished
interest or capacity for sex due to chronic disease. The discrimination
faced by gay people because of their sexual preference will be present
in the later years, perhaps even more so, since older people are generally less tolerant of those who are gay, and the general public does not
expect older people to be very sexually involved. There are some differences in the sexual accommodation to old age between gay elderly
and straight elderly but generally these differences are minor.

Some older people may discover that they prefer relationships with the same sex in their later years. Aging sometimes allows a latent homosexual or lesbian person to acknowledge that sexual preferences following the death or loss of the heterosexual partner. However, given the limited research on gay elderly, it is difficult to estimate how frequently such shifts in sexual preference occur in later life. In the later years, the preference for same sex relationships may not be overtly sexual, but may merely be a preference for the companionship of a person of the same sex. This choice may be made by persons who have a limited interest in sexual activity and who find that same sex companionship is a convenient way to avoid what, for them, may be the hassle of sexual activity. For many older adults, sexual health is not necessarily based on regular genital sexual activity; it is based more on the opportunity to be respected and regarded as sexual beings with their own manner of sexual preference, including sexual retirement if that is their choice.

Throughout their lives, most men and women establish companionable relationships with members of both sexes, even though sexual expression may have been limited to members of one sex. In old age, the imbalance in the numbers of the sexes caused by the greater life expectancy of women may complicate lifelong preferences of sexual activity. By age sixty-five, nearly one-half of the married women are already widowed. By age eighty-five, the ratio of women to men is nearly three to one. It is apparent to the heterosexual woman that the opportunities for maintaining lifelong heterosexual relationships are greatly reduced. This does not necessarily mean a sexless existence for the widowed woman. Bearing in mind that sexuality is something more than sexual intercourse, meaningful relationships may be established with new friends that meet many of the needs once filled by a spouse or lover. Of course some women will also be able to move on and build new courtships and relationships that are sexually fulfilling.

At any senior center or congregate meal site, the gathering of groups of women socially interacting with one another is commonplace. Many times men, although fewer in number, will also choose to spend their social time with each other. These gatherings are highly valued same sex relationships. The majority of these contacts are nonsexual in the narrow definition of the term but are nonetheless important to sexual health. Typically, such same sex companions will greet each other warmly with a hug and a kiss; they may hold hands or join arms while walking, and they will spend important and valued time together. The act of physical touch is somewhat less frequent with groups of older men, especially in our North American culture. In other parts of the world, men commonly embrace each other or walk hand in hand without others considering such activity to be homosexual. Given the realities of aging and the continued need for close communication with others, such same sex relationships contribute immensely to sexual health.

As sexual human beings, we remain sexual beings when we are with members of either sex. Throughout life we have learned to love members of both sexes, even though we may be sexually stimulated only by members of one sex—and then that sexual stimulation is often restricted to very few members of that sex, those with whom we have a deep love relationship. Again, this should not negate the importance of our sexual nature in all human relationships. To feel good, loved, and respected by a member of our same sex is part of sexual health. It reduces the loneliness in our lives and helps us cope with some of the sexual frustrations that the realities of aging may present in later life.

If we speak in terms of companionship rather than genital sexual activity, we will discover that most human beings are bisexual. We are capable of enjoying social contact with members of each sex and, depending upon the occasion and our needs, we will seek out the companionship of others according to their gender. Usually such relationships, including same sex relationships, are understood and accepted within the elderly community. With the exception perhaps of the situations described in the previous chapter, most family members are happy when their older relatives have good friends of the same sex available to them. In many cases, the family members may be even more comfortable if the widowed relative chooses someone of the same sex rather than a member of the opposite sex to be a close friend. As we have mentioned, same sex relationships for the nongay elderly may be a functional way of coping with voluntarily chosen sexual retirement. Same sex companions accept such relationships as essentially social rather than sexual.

Despite the absence of overt sexual contact, however, such relationships often contain many of the components of a sexual relationship. The success or failure of such relationships may be felt keenly. Illness or death of a same sex companion may be as traumatic as the death or illness of a spouse or a heterosexual partner. Jealousy may be present in such relationships, along with the vast array of other human emotions. Our sense of well-being and personal mental health is clearly affected by the successful flow of events associated with these relationships.

For professionals involved in providing health or social care to an older person, it is important to remain sensitive to the significance of same sex relationships in the life of an older person. This should include, of course, an awareness that some older people are gay. In taking a social or sexual history that covers the active sexuality of a client or patient, the professional should pay special attention to the possibility of same sex sexual relationships. It is dangerous to assume either that (1) older people are necessarily sexually retired, or that (2) if not sexually retired, they are only sexually active with a partner of the opposite sex. Appreciating the importance of same sex relationships in the lives of most older persons will help to reduce such oversights, especially in terms of understanding the gay community, the gay lifestyle, and the gay institutions upon which homosexual and lesbian individuals rely for support.

Gay elderly persons who are sexually active need to think through the meaning of aging with regard to sexual health. They must prepare themselves for the possibility of losing a sexual partner through illness or death, although this possibility is perhaps somewhat lessened by the fact that same sex partners will share the same life expectancy if they are approximately the same age. They must be knowledgeable about the effects of aging on their sexual interests and responsiveness, particularly if they have a chronic illness for which they are receiving treatment. They also face the issue of boredom and routine in their sexual lives, as do heterosexual couples. They may even have to face the possibility that their same sex partner may decide to retire sexually. Since most gay elderly have developed a rather marked independence over their lifetimes, the loss of social support because of the absence of children or distancing from close family may not be as traumatic as that which is often felt by straight elderly.

As we discussed earlier, our sexual nature is quite complicated and is constantly influenced by our mental state, as well as by our physical well-being. Often, especially in later life, we are faced with reevaluating and renegotiating our sexual relationships with another person. This is indeed a challenge, frustrating at times, but worth the investment of our energies. Sexual health is definitely a part of holistic health. A fully loved older person can accept a great deal of pain and loss. An older person who feels unloved is especially vulnerable to the vicissitudes of aging.

Many unanswered questions regarding the impact of aging in the gay elderly remain. Because homosexuality and lesbianism have been closeted, particularly in the current older generation, we cannot fully appreciate how the nuances of aging have affected the lifelong sexuality of the elderly gay population. We owe a great deal to the handful of researchers like Ray Berger who have had the courage and interest to explore this phenomenon. Sexual health for the gay elderly in old age cannot be fully explored until this field of investigation is researched further. Beyond this, we repeat our position that same sex relationships are important to both communities of elderly—the gays and the straights. This will become increasingly true if the life expectancies of men and women continue to be as disparate as they are today.

Although this is perhaps the shortest chapter in our book, it may well be the most important. In old age we apparently begin to spend more time with members of our same sex. In monitoring sexual health, we need to assure that such relationships are meaningful and, if and where possible, also sexually fulfilling. As we have repeatedly advised, sexual fulfillment does not imply that active genital sexual contact is required. It does imply, however, that the relationships themselves are fulfilling and serve the purpose of promoting the well-being of both partners.

Like professionals who serve the elderly, family members who are concerned about an older relative need to appreciate the importance of same sex relationships in the life of their relative. When family members live at some distance from their elderly relative, the most important supportive relationships may be those of friends and neighbors. Nurturing and supporting these relationships is perhaps the best support a family member can provide.

In ending this chapter, we would like to share the final paragraph from Raymond Berger's book, *Gay and Gray* (1982):

> If we look deeply into the lives of our respondents, we see a startling truth about the nature of preconceived categories into which we are so fond of placing ourselves and others. To the extent that each of us is a sexual being with needs for affection, there are no heterosexuals or homosexuals—there are only human beings with sexual and affectional needs to be fulfilled in a variety of ways. To the extent that each of us is a survivor of life, we are all aging. While we must not ignore real differences among people's ages and sexual needs, we must also be ready to challenge our preconceptions about the significance of these differences. (p. 202).

Appendix A
Key to the Adult Sexuality Knowledge and Attitude Test (ASKAT)

Please answer all questions. Circle T (true) or F (false) at the right. Do not answer as you *think* you should but as you really feel.

(The chapter numbers in parentheses indicate where the question is discussed. The asterisk indicates the correct answer.)

1. The majority of persons over age sixty-five have little capacity for sexual relations. (Chapter 1)　　　T　F*

2. People who have heart trouble should abstain from sexual activity because of the strain it puts on the heart. (Chapter 4)　　　T　F*

3. Illness rather than age is the usual reason why an older person stops having sexual relations. (Chapters 1, 2, 4, 6)　　　*T　F

4. Diabetes can cause impotence in males. (Chapter 4)　　　*T　F

5. The biological sexual drive in older men is considerably stronger than in older women. (Chapter 7)　　　T　F*

6. Changes in sexual interest and activity in women can often be caused by the loss of female hormones (estrogen) following menopause. (Chapter 3)   *T   F

7. Most women experience complicated physical and emotional symptoms with menopause. (Chapter 3)   T   F*

8. Most men experience a significant loss of male hormones with their "change of life." (Chapter 1)   T   F*

9. In the absence of regular sexual intercourse, the vagina of an older woman may shrink, shorten, and lose elasticity. (Chapters 3, 4, 5)   *T   F

10. Sexual feelings may remain for the older woman, but clitoral sexual sensations generally disappear by age sixty. (Chapter 3)   T   F*

11. Older women rarely masturbate. (Chapter 7)   T   F*

12. Regular sexual activity appears to stimulate hormone (estrogen) production in the postmenopausal woman. (Chapter 3)   *T   F

13. Since the clitoral area of older women becomes more sensitive, sexual partners need to take this into consideration during sexual relations. (Chapter 3)   *T   F

14. There is a significant decrease in the production of semen in the older male. (Chapter 3)   *T   F

15. Older men, unlike young men, often cannot have a follow-up erection/ejaculation within a short time after sexual intercourse. (Chapter 3)   *T   F

16. Male fertility (sperm production) usually ends by age sixty. (Chapter 5)   T   F*

17. Sexual activity is a good form of exercise therapy for the back, stomach, and pelvic muscles of older persons. (Chapter 4)   *T   F

18. Men with prostate problems may experience diminished sexual desires. (Chapters 4, 5)   *T   F

19. An older women who continues to be sexually active will probably not be able to experience an orgasm. (Chapter 3)   T   F*

20. Continued sexual activity by elderly men may lead to prostate problems. (Chapters 4, 5)   T   F*

21. Impotence in older men is an expected development in the aging process. (Chapter 3)   T   F*

22. Excessive alcohol intake in men may produce impotence. (Chapters 4, 5, 6)   *T   F

23. A hysterectomy inevitably produces physical changes that result in diminished sexual desire in women. (Chapters 5, 6)   T   F*

24. Tranquilizers, antidepressants, and certain antihypertensive drugs can cause loss of sexual desire in men and women. (Chapter 5)   *T   F

25. Toxic changes in the blood from nicotine may reduce sexual interest. (Chapter 4)   *T   F

26. Some postmenopausal women may experience an increased interest in sexual intercourse. (Chapters 3, 6)   *T   F

27. Healthy men over the age of sixty have greater control of ejaculation than do younger men. (Chapter 3)   *T   F

28. Widowhood is the most common cause of reduced sexual activity among older women. (Chapters 4, 9, 10)   *T   F

29. Physical changes in the vagina of the older woman reduce the likelihood of pain or discomfort with intercourse. (Chapter 3)   T   F*

30. The vagina of most older women is too fragile for frequent (that is, daily) sexual intercourse. (Chapter 3)   T   F*

31. A hysterectomy diminishes (or interferes with) a woman's ability to experience orgasm. (Chapter 3)   T   F*

32. Regular sexual activity is the best way to maintain sexual functioning in later life. (Chapters 2, 6)   *T   F

33. By age seventy most men are impotent. (Chapter 6)   *T   F

34. Older men are more likely to masturbate than are older women. (Chapter 7)   T   F*

35. A man in good health can continue to father children throughout his lifetime. (Chapter 5)   *T   F

36. Hot flashes and dizziness are unavoidable effects of menopause. (Chapter 3)   T   F*

37. In an older man, the penis softens quickly after ejaculation. (Chapter 3)   *T   F

38. The level of sexual interest and activity in old age generally parallels one's patterns of sexual interest and activity at a younger age. (Chapter 2)   *T   F

39. For many older people, the ability to perform sexually continues long after activity ceases. (Chapter 2)   *T   F

40. Older persons seldom have sexual fantasies or dreams. (Chapter 2)   T   F*

41. Masturbation is a common way for older persons to obtain sexual release. (Chapter 7)   *T   F

42. Older persons continue to be interested in sexual feelings (touch, kissing) but not in sexual intercourse. (Chapter 2)   T   F*

43. As a man ages, it takes longer for him to achieve an erection. (Chapter 3) *T F

44. Eating a big meal prior to sexual intercourse will stimulate sexual responsiveness in older persons. (Chapters 4, 7) T F*

45. A stroke is a frequent cause of impotence in men. (Chapter 4) T F*

46. Anemia may cause diminished sexual interest in older women. (Chapter 4) *T F

47. Sexual blushing (redness in the area of the abdomen and breasts) is less common in older women than in younger women. (Chapter 3) *T F

48. It is not uncommon for an older woman to experience some pain with orgasm. (Chapter 3) *T F

49. An older woman may experience shrinkage or atrophy of the vagina in the absence of regular sexual intercourse, making any resumption of intercourse initially painful. (Chapters 1, 3, 4, 5, 7) *T F

Please answer all questions. Remember, do not answer these as you think you should but as you really feel. Use the number that most closely describes the way you feel.

(1) Agree (2) Strongly Agree (3) Disagree (4) Strongly disagree

1. Masturbation by older persons is an acceptable method of relieving sexual tension. ( )

2. Old men should not be left alone with young female children for a long period of time. ( )

3. Sexual activity declines with age because of the loss of physical attractiveness of older men and women. ( )

4. Sexual contact between an elderly woman and a young man is improper. ( )

5. Unmarried people in nursing homes should not be permitted to have sex together, even if they request it. ( )

6. Oral-genital sexual activity at any age shows an excessive desire for physical pleasure. ( )

7. Elderly individuals should be encouraged to remain active sexually. ( )

8. Only people who are married to each other should have sexual intercourse. ( )

9. Premarital intercourse is much more common today than it was fifty years ago. ( )

10. Masturbation is an acceptable way to experience sexual pleasure. ( )

11. Sexual responsiveness is usually greater in women and men who have less education. ( )

12. Elderly couples should restrict their sexual activity to nighttime or to darkened rooms. ( )

13. Regular sexual functioning is important in later life for maintaining a sense of well-being. ( )

14. Married couples in nursing homes should have the freedom to engage in sexual intercourse, as long as it is in privacy. ( )

15. It is socially acceptable for an elderly unmarried man and an elderly unmarried woman to live together. ( )

16. Elderly persons with sexual problems should consult with their personal physician or a counselor. ( )

17. People remain sexual beings with needs and feelings throughout their lifetimes. ( )

Appendix B
Suggestions for
Further Reading

Blazer, D.G. *Depression in Late Life*. St. Louis, Mo.: C.V. Mosby, 1982.

Bowker, L.H. *Humanizing Institutions for the Aged*. Lexington, Mass.: Lexington Books, 1982.

Brecher, E.M., and the editors of Consumer Report Books. *Love, Sex and Aging*. Boston: Little, Brown, 1984.

Butler, R.N., and M.I. Lewis. *Aging and Mental Health: Positive Psychosocial and Biomedical Approaches*. St. Louis, Mo.: C.V. Mosby, 1982.

Comfort, A. *The Joy of Sex*. New York: Crown Publishers, 1972.

———. *Sexual Consequences of Disability*. Philadelphia: George F. Stickley, 1978.

———. *A Good Age*. New York: Simon and Schuster, 1979.

Crain, D.C. *The Arthritis Handbook: A Patient's Manual on Arthritis, Rheumatism and Gout*. Smithtown, N.Y.: Exposition Press, 1972.

Duvoisin, R.C. *Parkinson's disease: A Guide for Patient and Family*. New York: Raven Press, 1983.

Freeman, J.T. *Sexual Aspects of Aging: The Care of the Geriatric Patient*. St. Louis, Mo.: C.V. Mosby, 1971.

Gochros, H.L., and J. Fisher. *Treat Yourself to a Better Sex Life*. Englewood Cliffs, N.J.: Prentice-Hall, 1979.

Gordon, M. *Old Enough to Feel Better: A Medical Guide to Seniors*. Radner, Pa.: Chilton Bock Co. 1981.

Gross, L. *How Much Is Too Much? The Effects of Social Drinking*. New York: Random House, 1983.

Henig, R.M. *The Myth of Senility: Misconceptions about the Brain and Aging.* Garden City, N.Y. Doubleday, Anchor Books, 1981.

Kamen, B., and S. Kamen, *Osteoporosis: What It Is, How to Prevent It, How to Stop It.* New York: Pinnacle, 1984.

Kolodny, R.C., W.H. Masters, and V.E. Johnson *Geriatric Sexuality: Textbook of Sexual Medicine.* Boston: Little, Brown, 1979.

Kreis, B. *To Love Again: An Answer to Loneliness.* New York: Seabury Press, 1975.

Leslie, D.K., and J.W. McLure. *Exercises for the Elderly.* Iowa City, Iowa: University of Iowa, 1975.

Levitt, P.M., et al. *The Cancer Reference Book: Direct Answers to Everyone's Questions.* New York: Pennington Press, 1978.

Loewinsohn, R.J. *Survival Handbook for Widows (and for Relatives and Friends Who Want to Understand).* Published by American Association of Retired Persons. Glenview, Ill.: Scott, Foresman, 1984.

Mace, N.L., and P.V. Rabins. *The 36-Hour Day.* Baltimore: Johns Hopkins University Press, 1981.

Masters, W.H., and V.E. Johnson. *Human Sexual Response.* Boston: Little, Brown, 1966.

———. *Human Sexual Inadequacy.* Boston: Little, Brown, 1970.

Munjack, D.J., and L.J. Oziel. *Sexual Medicine and Counseling in Office Practice: A Comprehensive Treatment Guide.* Boston: Little, Brown, 1980.

Noteloritz, M., and M. Ware. *Stand Tall: The Informed Woman's Guide to Preventing Osteoporosis.* Gainesville, Fla.: Triad, 1982.

Pesman, C. and the editors of *Esquire. How a Man Ages.* New York: Ballantine Books, 1984.

Professional Self-Help Aids Catalog. Brookfield, Ill.: Fred Sammons, 1984. (Includes wheelchair accessories, safety and personal care products, and household utensils to aid in daily living.)

Rose, R.C., and R. Capildeo. *Stroke, the Facts.* New York: Oxford University Press, 1981.

Special Products for People with Special Needs. Pequannok, N.J.: Maddak, 1984. (A catalog similar to *Professional Self-Help Aids Catalog.)*

Starr, B.D., and M.B. Weiner. *Sex and Sexuality in the Mature Years.* New York: Stein and Day, 1981.

Weg, R.B., ed. *Sexuality in the Later Years.* Orlando, Fla.: Academic Press, 1983.

Wilson, J. *Sexpression: Improving Your Sexual Communication.* Englewood Cliffs, N.J.: Prentice-Hall, 1980.

The film *Rose by Any Other Name* is distributed and sold by:

Adelphi University Center on Aging
Garden City, N.Y. 11530
Telephone (516) 486-4530.

It may be rented for $15.50 plus UPS charges from:

Unviersity Film and Video
University of Minnesota
1313 5th St. S.E.
Minneapolis, MN 55414
Telephone (800) 847-8251.

Bibliography

Alport, G. *Becoming*. New Haven: Yale University Press, 1955.

Arthritis Foundation. *Living and Loving: Information about Sex*. Altanta, Ga.: Arthritis Foundation, 1982.

———. *Sjogren's Syndrome*. Medical Information Series. Atlanta, Ga.: Arthritis Foundation, 1985.

Benson, R.C., Jr. "An Updated Approach to Correcting Impotence in Elderly Men." *Geriatrics* 40 (1985): 87–102.

Berger, R.M. *Gay and Gray: The Older Homosexual Man*. Urbana, Ill.: University of Illinois Press, 1982.

Bray, G.P., R.S. DeFrank, and T.L. Wolfe. "Sexual Functioning in Stroke Survivors." *Archives of Physical Medicine and Rehabilitation* 62 (1981): 286–88.

Burkhalter, P.K. "Sexuality and the cancer patient." In *Dynamics of Oncology Nursing*, edited by P.K. Burkhalter and D.L. Donley, 249–75. New York: McGraw-Hill, 1978.

Butler, R.N., and M.I. Lewis. *Sex after Sixty: A Guide for Men and Women for Their Later Years*. New York: Harper & Row, 1976.

Cochrane, M. "Immaculate infection." *Nursing Times* (26 September 1984): 31–32.

Curb, J.D., et al. "Long-Term Surveillance for Adverse Effects of Antihypertensive Drugs." *Journal of the American Medical Association* 253 (1985): 3263–68.

Dean, S.R. "Geriatric Sexuality: Normal, Needed, and Neglected." *Geriatrics* 29 (1974): 134–37.

Ellenberg, M. "Sexual Function in Diabetic Patients." *Annals of Internal Medicine* 92, part 2 (1980): 331–33.

Federal Register. *Skilled Nursing Facilities.* Washington, D.C.: Department of Health, Education, and Welfare, 39(193), part 2, October 3, 1974. Quoted in Wharton, G.F., III. *Sexuality and Aging: An Annotated Bibliography.* Metuchen, N.J.: Scarecrow Press, 1981.

Feinberg, T., and B. Goodman. "Affective Illness, Dementia, and Pseudodementia." *Clinical Psychiatry* 45 (1984): 99–103.

Fisher, I., and B. Lane. *The Widow's Guide to Life.* Englewood Cliffs, N.J.: Prentice-Hall, 1981.

Fletcher, E.C., and R.J. Martin. "Sexual Dysfunction and Erectile Impotence in Chronic Obstructive Pulmonary Disease." *Chest* 81 (1982): 413–21.

Gupta, M.C., and M.M. Singh. "Postinfarction Sexual Activity." *Journal of the Indian Medical Association* 79 (1981): 45–48.

Haugland, S. *Lecture Outline on Alcoholism/Chemical Dependency.* Des Moines, Iowa: Iowa Methodist Medical Center, 1985.

"Health Update: Blood Pressure Control without Heartache." *Better Homes and Gardens* (Sept. 1986): 71.

Masters, W.H., V.E. Johnson, and R.C. Kolodny. *Masters and Johnson on Sex and Human Loving.* Boston: Little, Brown, 1986.

Medical Economics Company. *Physicians' Desk Reference.* Oradell, N.J.: Jack E. Angel, 1986.

——. *Self-Medication: A Guide to Over-the-Counter Health Care Products.* Oradell, N.J.: Edward Barnhart, 1984.

National Institute on Aging Task Force. "Senility Reconsidered. Treatment Possibilities for Mental Impairment in the Elderly." *Journal of the American Medical Association* 244 (1980): 259–63.

National Institutes of Health. *Radiation Therapy and You: A Guide to Self-Help during Treatment.* National Institutes of Health Publication No. 85-2227. Bethesda, Md.: National Cancer Institute, 1985.

Renshaw, D.C. "Sexual Problems in Old Age, Illness, and Disability." *Psychosomatics* 22 (1981): 975–85.,

Sarna, T.P. "Concepts in Nursing Management of Patients Receiving Cancer Chemotherapy and Immunotherapy." In *Concepts of Oncology Nursing*, edited by D.L. Vredevoe et al., 81–150. Englewood Cliffs, N.J.: Prentice-Hall, 1981.

Scheingold, L.D., and N.W. Wagner. *Sound Sex and the Aging Heart.* New York: Human Sciences Press, 1974.

Smith, P.J., and R.L. Talbert. "Therapy Reviews. Sexual Dysfunction with Antihypertensive and Antipsychotic Agents." *Clinical Pharmacy* 5 (1986): 373–84.

Spark, R., R. White, and P. Connolly. "Impotence Is Not Always Psychogenic." *Journal of the American Medical Association* 243 (1980): 750–54.

United Scleroderma Foundation. *Sexuality and Scleroderma.* Watsonville, Calif.: United Scleroderma Foundation, 1983.

Walz, T.H., and N.S. Blum. *Adult Sexuality Knowledge and Attitude Test.* Iowa City, Iowa: University of Iowa, 1986.

Wharton, G.F., III. *Sexuality and Aging: An Annotated Bibliography.* Metuchen, N.J.: Scarecrow Press, 1981.

Yasko. J.M. "Sexual Dysfunction." In *Care of the Client Receiving External Radiation Therapy,* 192–201. Reston, Va.: Reston Publishing Company, 1982.

Index

About the Authors

Thomas H. Walz is a professor of social work and is former director of the Iowa Multidisciplinary Gerontology Center at the University of Iowa. He is a past president of the Mid-America Congress on Aging.

Nancee S. Blum is a medical writer and editor, and is a research assistant in the Department of Psychiatry at the University of Iowa. She has completed a certificate in aging studies and is currently enrolled in the Master's program in social work at the University of Iowa.